Tobias Warnken

Comparison of various methods for quantification of equine insulin under clinical settings for assessment of insulin dysregulation

Cuvillier Verlag Göttingen
Internationaler wissenschaftlicher Fachverlag

Bibliografische Information der Deutschen Nationalbibliothek

Die Deutsche Nationalbibliothek verzeichnet diese Publikation in der Deutschen Nationalbibliografie; detaillierte bibliographische Daten sind im Internet über http://dnb.d-nb.de abrufbar.

1. Aufl. - Göttingen: Cuvillier, 2019

Zugl.: Hannover (TiHo), Univ., Diss., 2019

© CUVILLIER VERLAG, Göttingen 2019

Nonnenstieg 8, 37075 Göttingen

Telefon: 0551-54724-0

Telefax: 0551-54724-21

www.cuvillier.de

ISBN 978-3-7369-7124-0

eISBN 978-3-7369-6124-1

University of Veterinary Medicine Hannover

Comparison of various methods for quantification of equine insulin under clinical settings for assessment of insulin dysregulation

Inaugural-Dissertation
to obtain the academic degree
Doctor medicinae veterinariae
(Dr. med. vet.)

submitted by
Tobias Warnken
Bremen

Hannover 2019

Academic supervision: **Prof. Dr. med. vet. Karsten Feige**

Clinic for Horses, University of Veterinary Medicine Hannover, Foundation, Hannover, Germany

Prof. Dr. med. vet. Korinna Huber

Institute of Animal Science, Faculty of Agricultural Sciences, University of Hohenheim, Stuttgart, Germany

1St Referee: **Prof. Dr. med. vet. Karsten Feige**

Prof. Dr. med. vet. Korinna Huber

2nd Referee: **Prof. Dr. Jürgen Rehage**

Clinic for Cattle, University of Veterinary Medicine Hannover, Foundation, Hannover, Germany

Day of the oral examination: 07.11.2019

Boehringer Ingelheim Vetmedica GmbH financially supported a part of this research.

Parts of the thesis have been published previously or communicated:

Publications in *peer-reviewed* journals:

Warnken T, Huber K, Feige K: **Comparison of three different methods for quantification of equine insulin.** *BMC Vet Res. 2016; 12(1): 196.*

Warnken T, Delarocque J, Schumacher S, Huber K, Feige K: **Retrospective analysis of insulin responses to standard dosed oral glucose tests (OGTs) via naso-gastric tubing towards definition of an objective cut-off.** *Acta Vet Scand; 2018;60(1):4.*

Presentations at conferences:

Warnken T, Huber K, Feige K (2016) **Comparison and clinical applicability of three methods for measurement of equine insulin.** InnLab 2016, Berlin 29.-30.01.2016

Warnken T, Huber K, Feige K (2017) **Comparison and clinical interpretation of three methods for measurement of equine insulin.** Dorothy Russell Havemeyer International Equine Endocrinology Summit, Miami, 03.-07.01.2017.

Warnken T, Schmicke M, Huber K, Feige K (2018) **Selection of assay for quantification of equine insulin affects results of oral glucose test and combined glucose-insulin test in horses.** 11th ECEIM Congress 2018, Ghent 09.11.-10.11.2018.

Warnken T, Schmicke M, Huber K, Feige K (2018) **Selection of assay for quantification of equine insulin affects results of oral glucose test and combined glucose-insulin test in horses.** ACVIM Forum 2019, Phoenix 06.06.-08.06.2019.

FÜR OPA

TABLE OF CONTENTS

ABBREVIATIONS

ACTH	adrenocorticotropic hormone
ANOVA	analysis of variance
BCS	body condition score
BW	body weight
CGIT	combined glucose-insulin test
CLIA	chemiluminescence immunoassay
CV	coefficient of variation
EIA	enzyme immuno assay
ELISA	enzyme-linked immunosorbent assay
EMS	equine metabolic syndrome
FIG	figure
g	gram
HEC	hyperinsulinemic euglycemic clamp
HPLC	high performance liquid chromatography
ID	insulin dysregulation
IR	insulin resistance
IRMA	immunoradiometric assay
IU	international units
IV	intravenous
IQR	interquartile range
kDa	kilo Dalton
kg	kilogram
LLOD	lower limit of detection

MetS	metabolic syndrome (human)
mg	milligram
min	minutes
mL	milliliter
MS	mass spectrometry
μIU	micro international units
NGT	naso-gastric tube
NSC	non-structural carbohydrates
OGT	oral glucose test
OST	oral sugar test
PO	per os
PPID	pituitary *pars intermedia* dysfunction
RIA	radioimmunoassay
RM	repeated measures
RUD	recovery upon dilution
SD	standard deviation
SVD	singular value decomposition
TAB	table

1 INTRODUCTION

Metabolic pathologies, obesity and endocrinopathies play an increasingly significant role in equine veterinary medicine. The prevalence of obesity is high in the equine population with rates ranging between 30 to 48 % (Thatcher et al. 2008; Wyse et al. 2008; Giles et al. 2014). In addition, horses presented to a first opinion hospital for evaluation of laminitis were hyperinsulinemic in 66 % of the cases (Karikoski et al. 2011), indicating the outstanding clinical importance. Impaired insulin regulation reflected by hyperinsulinemia and caused by insulin dysregulation (ID) and/or insulin resistance (IR) is a common feature in equine endocrinopathies with partially severe and life-threating consequences for the individual affected. The assessment of ID or IR by dynamic challenge tests can be difficult under clinical conditions based on complex and time-consuming testing procedures but provides advantages compared to solely analyses of resting insulin and glucose concentrations. Nevertheless, in addition to complex diagnostic testing protocols, most test procedures require analyses of equine insulin in blood samples collected either during or after these dynamic stimulation tests. Quantification of equine insulin is provided by several specialized laboratories using varying immunoassays. However, analyses of basal samples or samples obtained during dynamic diagnostic procedures might require variable laboratory and immunoassay demands for exact quantification of equine insulin. Moreover, reliable references ranges for the combination of commonly used diagnostic procedures, for example, the oral glucose test (OGT) performed via nasogastric tubing (NGT), and analyses with specific immunoassays are lacking.

2 LITERATURE REVIEW

2.1 INSULIN DYSREGULATION

Glucose homeostasis is tightly controlled in physiological conditions to maintain essential metabolic homeostasis of the organism. Imbalances in insulin regulation can occur under either physiological conditions, such as pregnancy and lactation with redistribution of energy sources (Fowden et al. 1984; Maresh 2001), or pathophysiological conditions. The term ID describes impaired regulation in this complex system. The ID can be reflected by basal hyperinsulinemia, excessive or prolonged postprandial hyperinsulinemia and/or by IR (Frank and Tadros 2014; Bertin and De Laat 2017; Durham et al. 2019). The IR is defined as the inability of tissues to respond adequately to insulin (Muniyappa et al. 2008). It can be reflected by a decreased insulin sensitivity, which is characterized by a normal maximal biological effect combined with a need for an increased insulin concentration to achieve this maximal biological effect. By contrast, a decreased insulin responsiveness is characterized by a decreased maximal biological effect combined with normal insulin concentrations (Kahn 1978; De Koster and Opsomer 2013). Underlying pathomechanisms of IR have not been identified completely in humans nor in various animal species. However, several hypotheses have been postulated, including a reduced number of insulin receptors in target tissues due to downregulation, receptor dysfunction or disturbed post receptor signaling (Kahn 1980; Shanik et al. 2008). Horses severely affected by IR have typically increased basal insulin concentrations. However, mild cases may not stand out with basal hyperinsulinemia. This hyperinsulinemia can be symptomatic of tissue IR when it occurs as a compensatory response to peripheral tissue IR. In contrast to the situations in humans, horses normally compensate for reduced insulin sensitivity and develop hyperinsulinemia concurrent with normoglycemia, whereas humans suffer from hyperinsulinemia and hyperglycemia (Divers 2008). However, recent research highlighted the fact that ID can occur independently of tissue IR, reflected by increased insulinemic responses of ponies to PO-applied glucose compared to IV-applied glucose (De Laat et al. 2016a). It was suggested that the hyperinsulinemia is not just a sequela of IR and that the enteroinsular axis might contribute to ID with intensified insulin secretion mediated by incretine stimulation. Impaired secretion and the action of glucagon-like peptide 1 as one incretine has been identified in humans suffering from diabetes mellitus type II (Toft-Nielsen et al. 2001a) and intravenous glucagon-like peptide 1 infusion lowered plasma glucose in diabetes type II patients (Toft-Nielsen et al. 2001b). Glucagon-like peptide 1 has been analyzed in horses and positively correlated with postprandial insulin concentrations in healthy and in insulin-dysregulated horses after glycemic challenges (Bamford et al. 2015; De Laat et al. 2016a). The hypothesis of impaired action of the enteroinsulinar axis is further supported by several studies reporting weak to missing correlation between direct and indirect measures of tissue IR using enteral glycemic stimulations and, therefore, testing more diverse aspects of ID (Pratt et al. 2005: Banse and Mcfarlane 2014; Pratt-Phillips et al. 2015; Dunbar et al. 2016). However, recent studies were not able to identify differences in incretine concentrations between healthy insulin-sensitive and insulin-dysregulated horses after an oral glycemic challenge test (Chameroy et al. 2016) and healthy and insulin-dysregulated ponies after grazing pasture (Fitzgerald et al. 2019b).

2.1.1 ASSOCIATED EQUINE DISEASES

2.1.1.1 EQUINE METABOLIC SYNDROME

The Equine Metabolic Syndrome (EMS) is more of a collection of risk factors and a symptom complex than an actual disease and is a rising concern in the equine population (Durham et al. 2019). The term EMS was first introduced into veterinary medicine by Johnson (2002) and referred to a cluster of clinical signs predisposing horses and ponies for the development of laminitis. The term and the characteristics were adopted from human medicine where the Human Metabolic Syndrome (MetS) describes a disease pattern in which obesity, diabetes type II and cardiovascular diseases are the major symptoms. Similar symptoms in equids compared to the situation in human medicine had been observed. Generalized obesity or regional

4

accumulation of fat are frequently observed in affected horses (Treiber et al. 2006; Carter et al. 2009; Giles et al. 2015; Fitzgerald et al. 2019a). The lean EMS phenotype has been described more recently and is increasingly perceived (Durham et al. 2019). A predisposition to laminitis has the major significance, together with obesity. A laboratory key finding and essential for the confirmation of the diagnosis of EMS is the accompanying ID (Frank et al. 2010; Frank and Tadros 2014; Bertin and De Laat 2017; Equine Endocrinology Group 2018; Durham et al. 2019). Additional clinical conditions associated with EMS include hypertriglyceridemia or dyslipidemia (Frank et al. 2006; Treiber et al. 2006; Carter et al. 2009), hyperleptinemia (Cartmill et al. 2003), hypoadiponectemia (Menzies-Gow et al. 2017) and cardiovascular changes, including arterial hypertension (Bailey et al. 2008), and myocardial changes (Heliczer et al. 2017). Altered reproductive cycling in mares (Vick et al. 2006) and generally increased proinflammatory markers (Vick et al. 2007) are further clinical findings being discussed in the context of EMS. In general, EMS seems to occur more commonly in physically inactive and overfed horses and anecdotally in certain native breeds which exhibit the obese, EMS-like phenotype more commonly (Durham et al. 2019). Recent research highlights a possible inherited predisposition for EMS in some breeds, partially based on the assumption that these breeds had genetically adapted to survival under suboptimal nutritional conditions (McCue et al. 2015; Lewis et al. 2017). Interestingly, further studies investigated genetics in EMS horses providing evidence for potential genetic predisposition (Norton et al. 2019a, 2019b).

2.1.1.2 PITUITARY *PARS INTERMEDIA* DYSFUNCTION

Pituitary *pars intermedia* dysfunction (PPID), previously known as Equine Cushing Syndrome, is a severe neuroendocrine equine disease associated with metabolic perturbations and even impaired insulin regulation in some cases (Equine Endocrinology Group 2017). Affected horses are normally over 15 years of age and recent studies have reported prevalence rates of up to 30 % for horses over 15 years (McFarlane 2011). Affected horses generally show clinical signs such as regional adiposity, with atypical adipose tissue accumulation in the neck and tailhead region.

Hirsutism or hypertrichosis is the most unique and frequent clinical sign in horses suffering from PPID occurring in 55 to 80 % of cases. Further clinical signs include polyuria together with polydipsia and concurrent muscle atrophy resulting in poor body condition in some cases (Schott 2002; McFarlane 2011). The underlying etiology of PPID is a specific expansion of the melanotrophic cells of the *pars intermedia* of the pituitary gland (McFarlane and Cribb 2005). The hyperplasia of the *pars intermedia* of the pituitary gland is based on a loss of dopaminergic inhibition by the hypothalamus and uncontrolled release of POMC, mainly adrenocorticotropic hormone (ACTH) (McFarlane 2011). The underlying mechanism for the lack of dopaminergic control is not known. However, there are suggestions that oxidative stress may play a significant role and may led to neurodegeneration (McFarlane and Cribb 2005). Interestingly, some horses with PPID develop mild to severe ID. Studies reporting ranges of 30 to 60 % of PPID horses also being diagnosed with ID (Schott 2002; McFarlane 2011; McGowan et al. 2013; Mastro et al. 2015). The exact potential cross-link between disturbed cortisol regulation and the occurrence of ID is not fully understood. However, the concurrent ID is discussed to dramatically increase the risk of the development of endocrinopathic laminitis in PPID cases which are already being treated with pergolide mesylate.

2.1.2 ENDOCRINOPATHIC LAMINITIS

Laminitis is a life-threatening disease of horses and ponies causing acute or chronic painful conditions of the hooves (Pollitt 2004). It often results in acute or chronic lameness in affected equids, frequently necessitating euthanasia due to welfare aspects. Laminitis is defined as a failure of the laminar tissue of the hooves' lamellar-distal phalangeal attachment apparatus (Pollitt 1996, 2004). Unfortunately, the exact pathomechanisms are still unknown in their entirety despite an excessive research effort. Several etiologies of laminitis have been described and postulated, for example, alimentary and inflammatory induction (Garner et al. 1975; Galey et al. 1991; Van Eps and Pollitt 2006; Pollitt and Visser 2010). However, the etiology of laminitis may be multifactorial in different conditions and is often a result of several systemic disease entities. Despite well-known causes of laminitis development, such as, endotoxemia or overweight bearing, there is growing evidence of an association with endocrine dysfunction (McGowan 2008, 2010; Patterson-Kane et al. 2018; De Laat 2019). Donaldson et al. (2004) reported the prevalence of PPID defined by a single high plasma ACTH concentration in around 70 % of laminitis cases. Moreover, Karikoski et al. (2011) reported evidence of an endocrinopathy in 89 % of admitted cases presented to a first opinion hospital for evaluation of laminitis. A diagnosis of PPID was made in 33 % of cases, whereas hyperinsulinemia was present in 66 % of cases (Karikoski et al. 2011). Consistent with these findings, De Laat et al. (2019) reported that horses and ponies suffering from laminitis with concurrent endocrinopathies have more marked hyperinsulinemia and that higher basal insulin concentrations in these cases were associated with more severe lameness. In addition, several studies identified elevated serum insulin concentrations as a risk factor for the development of laminitis (Carter et al. 2009; Menzies-Gow et al. 2017). Multiple experimental studies have been performed to prove the relationship between insulin and laminitis in which laminitis was induced under hyperinsulinemic conditions. Prolonged IV infusion of insulin by hyperinsulinemic euglycemic clamps induced clinical laminitis and histopathological changes in the hooves in previously healthy ponies (Asplin et al. 2007, Asplin et al. 2010). Additionally, De Laat et al. (2010) induced laminitis in healthy Standardbred horses within 48 h by prolonged hyperinsulinemia, proving insulin-mediated induction of laminitis even in more insulin-sensitive breeds. Despite the fact that artificial exogenous hyperinsulinemia induced laminitis, De Laat et al. (2012), furthermore, showed that prolonged IV glucose infusions provoking constant endogenous hyperinsulinemia were also able to induce histopathological lamellar changes consistent with laminitis. Despite studies focusing on artificial hyperinsulinemia provoked by IV infusion of exogenous insulin or glucose, Meier et al. (2017) showed the direct link between a pathologically high postprandial insulin response and the occurrence of experimentally induced laminitis by a dietary challenge high in nonstructural carbohydrates (NSC).

2.1.3 ASSESSMENT OF INSULIN DYSREGULATION IN HORSES

Several diagnostic procedures are currently routinely used for the assessment of disturbed insulin regulation in equids. However, different test procedures provide diverse information regarding the aspects of ID. Basal measures of either insulin or combinations of glucose and insulin allow the detection of severe basal hyperinsulinemia but may lack identifying cases with inconspicuous basal insulin and exacerbated postprandial insulin concentrations in response to carbohydrate ingestion. Olley et al. (2019), for example, identified a poor sensitivity of fasted insulin concentrations at conventional cutoff values compared to the IV combined glucose-insulin test. However, studies comparing basal insulin concentrations and results from PO testing are not currently available.

Therefore, dynamic diagnostic tests assessing the horse's response to a glycemic stimulation are currently recommended for the assessment of ID (Bertin and De Laat 2017; Equine Endocrinology Group 2018; Durham et al. 2019). Variable standardized OGT protocols have been established. Based on the physiological mode of action, OGTs are recommended to assess pathological postprandial hyperinsulinemia (Equine Endocrinology Group 2018; Durham et al. 2019). In-feed OGTs can be performed and may offer the most physiological test principle by measuring insulin and glucose response following the ingestion of a meal artificially enriched with NSC, such as glucose or dextrose powder (De Laat et al. 2016a; Smith et al. 2016; Bertin and De Laat 2017; De Laat and Sillence 2017; Meier et al. 2017). The dextrose or glucose dosage for implementation ranges from 0.5 to 1 g/kg bodyweight (BW) (Frank et al. 2010; Frank and Geor 2014; Durham et al. 2019). A clinical decision can be made based on several cutoff values reported in literature. However, the variable cutoff values or reference ranges have to be used based on the glucose dose implemented and the selection of the immunoassay used for the analysis of the equine insulin (Frank and Tadros 2014; Durham et al. 2019). Despite variable dosages and cutoff values, the repeatability of this test procedure is crucial and horses and ponies often refuse to ingest the complete ratio or need variable times for complete ingestion and, therefore, preclude the reliable diagnosis of ID (De Laat and Sillence 2017).

Schuver et al. (2014) described the Oral Sugar Test as a simplified test to assess the insulin response after a defined NSC challenge. Commercially available corn syrup (Karo Corn Syrup®, ACH Food Companies Inc., Memphis, Tennessee, USA) is administered PO for test implementation. The dosages described range from 0.15 ml/kg BW (Schuver et al. 2014) to a recently suggested and recommended 0.45 ml/kg BW (Jocelyn et al. 2018). As a result of the dose comparison studies and further investigations, it was highlighted that increased amounts of corn syrup increase the diagnostic accuracy to assess ID (Manfredi 2016; Jacob et al. 2018a; Jocelyn et al. 2018). However, administration of increased amounts of corn syrup complicates the simple PO application procedure.

Variable reference ranges and cutoff values have been reported based on small numbers of the animals included and use of variable immunoassays, thus, often complicating diagnosing ID based on this test protocol in clinical practice. Diagnostic uncertainty might further occur due to variable composition of the syrup. Multiple analyses indicated controversial results regarding the ingredients and reported marked differences between different lots (Schuver et al. 2014; Jocelyn et al. 2018).

However, OGT can also be performed by glucose application via an NGT and provides the substantial benefit that an exact amount of glucose is administered within a specific period directly into the stomach of the animal tested (Ralston 2002). Although NGT may require trained veterinary personal and is an invasive procedure for diagnostic purposes, it might be the most standardized procedure and is often used in clinical routine when horses refuse to ingest the meal during in-feed OGTs. Nevertheless, there are no reliable cutoff values for the OGT via NGT and, therefore, cutoff values or reference ranges were adopted from different test protocols regardless of the underlying differences in their physiological mode of action and the immunoassay method used for quantification of equine insulin.

2.1.4 ASSESSMENT OF INSULIN RESISTANCE IN HORSES

Despite the assessment of basal hyperinsulinemia or pathologically high postprandial hyperinsulinemia as aspects of ID, assessment of tissue IR as another part of ID can be performed and achieved by several further test procedures. Measuring responses to IV administered insulin and/or glucose focus on the assessment of peripheral tissue insulin sensitivity and β-cell responsiveness. Tests such as the frequently sampled IV glucose tolerance test (Hoffman et al. 2003; Bailey et al. 2007; Durham et al. 2009) and the hyperinsulinemic euglycemic clamp (Pratt et al. 2005; Pratt-Phillips et al. 2015) are often used to investigate insulin and glucose regulation in experimental and research settings but are too complex and costly for routine clinical use. A simplified procedure such as the combined glucose-insulin test is a more practicable test in routine clinical use and is considered a direct method to assess tissue IR (Eiler et al. 2005). The capacity of the exogenous insulin to shift the injected glucose into the insulin-sensitive tissues is assessed by injection of 150 mg/kg BW glucose followed by an immediately injection of 0.1 IU/kg BW insulin. Whereas glucose concentration is monitored for 45 min, insulin is measured prior to injection and after 45 min. Insulin-sensitive horses show a typical two-phase blood glucose curve with an initial hyperglycemia followed by a second phase with hypoglycemia in which glucose concentrations drop below the initially determined baseline concentration. The first positive phase in insulin-resistant horses is prolonged due to a slower return to baseline. The 45-min value is used as a clinical cutoff value to distinguish between insulin-sensitive and -resistant individuals. Horses should achieve normal glucose concentrations and return to baseline levels within 45 minutes and insulin concentration should remain under 100 µIU/mL if insulin analysis is performed with a human-specific radioimmunoassay (RIA; Coat-A-Count, Diagnostic Products Corp, Los Angeles, California, USA; Eiler et al. 2005). Horses with insulin concentrations above 100 µIU/mL are secreting more insulin than normal or clearing the hormone from the circulation at a slower rate. Therefore, values above this range are interpreted as an indication of reduced insulin sensitivity (Eiler et al. 2005).

2.2 INSULIN

Insulin is the principal important hormone in the regulation of blood glucose homeostasis and essential for the organism's metabolic function (Wilcox 2005, Berg et al. 2018). Insulin is the main anabolic hormone and released after food intake in response to a rise in blood glucose concentration (Berg et al. 2018). Insulin's basic action is to promote the cellular uptake of glucose, fatty acids and amino acids and to initiate their further conversion into carbohydrate, fat and protein in insulin-dependent tissues (Wilcox 2005, Berg et al. 2018). Insulin is synthesized as the prohormone pre-proinsulin in the rough endoplasmic reticulum by the β-cells within the islets of Langerhans of the pancreas (Wilcox 2005). Pre-proinsulin consists of an A-chain and a B-chain coupled by a connecting peptide (C-peptide) (Conlon 2001). During translation in the rough endoplasmic reticulum, a single sequence of the pre-prohormone, the N-terminal sequence, is removed by proteases, resulting in proinsulin (Wilcox 2005, Berg et al. 2018). The proinsulin is transported to the Golgi apparatus, where proinsulin hexamers are formed (Steiner 2004). Finally, C-peptide is removed by enzymes during secretion of the proinsulin vesicle from the Golgi apparatus, resulting in the formation of insulin (Conlon 2001, Berg et al. 2018). Both proinsulin and insulin are secreted into the circulation but proinsulin has only a very limited biological activity compared to insulin (Wilcox 2005). The amino acid composition of insulin is highly conserved among many vertebrate species and was first characterized in humans by Fred Sanger (Stretton 2002). In addition to the highly conserved amino acid sequence, the positions of the disulfide bonds are the same for most species. These similarities lead to a three-dimensional conformation of insulin that is very similar across species (Conlon 2001). Thus, insulin from one species is often biologically active in other species, for which reason animal insulin was initially used for treatment of diabetes in men. Furthermore, there is a structural homology of insulin with insulin-like growth factors 1 and 2 (Yakar et al. 2000). Despite the highly conserved amino acid sequence of insulin, some slight differences between species exist and provoke changes of specific segments of the molecule. The equine insulin has a lower molecular weight of 5.748 kDa compared to human insulin with a molecular weight of 5.808 kDa and differs in the amino acid composition compared to human insulin at residues A-9 and B-30 (Ho et al. 2008; Kuuranne et al. 2008; Ho et al. 2011). The equine insulin molecule at residue A-9 consists of a glycine instead of a serine and at residue B-30, it consists of an alanine instead of a threonine in human insulin (Ho et al. 2008). The insulin is secreted in equimolar amounts with C-peptide into the circulation during exocytosis (Wilcox 2005). Insulin is produced and stored as a hexamer structure. Insulin in humans is cleared by liver tissue during the first pass effect from the portal vein for approximately 80 % (Meier et al. 2005) and circulating insulin is cleared mainly by glomerular filtration (Rabkin et al. 1984). Recent investigations in horses indicated hepatic clearance rates of approximately 30 % under basal conditions and approximately 60 % under infusion of dextrose (De Laat et al. 2016b). In contrast to insulin, C-peptide is predominantly extracted by the kidneys and does not undergo the first pass effect in the liver (Rabkin et al. 1984). When secreted into the blood stream, insulin binds to the insulin receptor in insulin-dependent and -sensitive tissues and initiates insulin-mediated glucose uptake by activation of insulin signaling (Saltiel and Kahn 2001). Insulin-mediated activation of insulin signaling was partially investigated in horses (Urschel et al. 2014b, 2014a) and indicated tissues' specific variations under hyperinsulinemic and hyperglycemic conditions (Warnken et al. 2017).

2.3 QUANTIFICATION OF INSULIN

Measurement of human insulin was first performed in 1959 by use of an RIA by Yalow and Berson (1959). Nowadays, immunoassay-based methods are used frequently in human and veterinary medicine for analyses of various analytes including hormones. The test principle is based on antigen-antibody reactions (Wild 2013). Thus, immunoassays can be used to analyze either antigens or antibodies based on the following reaction:

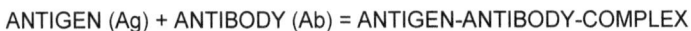

ANTIGEN (Ag) + ANTIBODY (Ab) = ANTIGEN-ANTIBODY-COMPLEX

Immunoassays can be generally grouped as competitive or non-competitive assays. Competitive assays are based on a defined and limited number of bindings sites of a protein (Ag) and a limited amount of a labelled ligand (Ab) (Giraudi et al. 1999, Davies 2013, Wild 2013). Thus, a competitive interaction between the labelled ligand and the unlabeled ligand from the sample analyzed occurs to bind on a defined and limited amount of an antibody. Based on the detection of the labelled ligand, the concentration of antigen-antibody complexes can be measured (Davies 2013). According to the fact that the labelled ligand is bound to the not-analyte-bound binding sites, the concentration of the analyte of interest is inversely proportional to the concentration of the antigen-antibody complexes. Competitive assays are not particularly suitable for the detection of very low concentrations of analytes compared to non-competitive assays, based on the fact that very low concentrations of the analyte are difficult to differentiate from the zero standard or calibrator (Giraudi et al. 1999). Non-competitive assays are usually solid-phase assays (Friemel 1991). The most common technique is the sandwich technique (Porstmann and Porstmann 1991), based on an immobilized antibody bound onto a microplate surface capturing the specific test analyte from the sample. After the incubation and binding process of the antibodies and the analyte, the unbound analyte and the remaining sample matrix are removed by a washing step. In a second step, another specifically labeled detection antibody is added and binds to free epitopes of the analyte to label it. Thus, the amount of analyte-bound binding sites labelled by the second antibody are detected in this technique (Davies 2013, Aydin 2015). In addition, the doubled binding by two specific antibodies increases the assay's specificity. Labeling might be achieved with radioactive isotopes (also called tracers) or enzyme-labeled markers providing a basis for a signal generation system. The signal generated can be radioactive with γ- or β-radiation or can be based on a color change, a fluorescent signal or a luminescent signal which can be measured and detected (Weeks et al. 2013).

Several immunoassay methods for the quantification of insulin have been developed since the initial RIA was designed and are commercially available for quantification of either human insulin or insulin in some animal species; mainly laboratory animals. Radioimmunoassays are based on radioactive-labeled antibodies that form a complex with the specific substrate (Skelly et al. 1973, Goldsmith 1975, Weeks et al. 2013). Radioactive iodine can be used as a tracer and iodine[125] and iodine[131] (radioactive isotopes) are used most frequently (Kunkel 1991, Weeks et al. 2013). The advantages of these tracers are their small sizes and, therefore, their negligible influence on the concurrent operating immune reaction in combination with the high traceability of even very low amounts and the low susceptibility to failure based on interference with biological substances in the sample matrix (Kunkel 1991, Weeks et al. 2013). Radioimmunoassays can be further divided into direct or indirect methods. In direct methods, the samples with the unlabeled antigen are incubated with the first antibody in the presence of the second antibody, which is labeled with a radioactive marker, such as iodine[125]. After incubation, the sample content is rinsed to remove unbound ^{125}I-labeled antibodies. Finally, the amount of bound and radioactive-labeled antigen-antibody complexes is then determined in a gamma counter. The concentration of the analyte in the samples in this technique is directly proportional to the radioactivity generated by the labeled antigen-antibody complexes. This kind of radiometric assay is called an immunoradiometric assay (IRMA) (Praither et al. 1985, Davies 2013). By contrast, indirect methods are based on the incubation of a fixed concentration of radioactive-labeled antigen with a constant dilution of antiserum, such that the concentration of antigen-binding sites on the antibody is limited (Davies 2013). If the sample and, thereby, unlabeled antigen is added to this system, there is competition between the labeled tracer and unlabeled antigen from the sample for the limited and constant number of binding sites on the antibody. Thus, the amount of radioactive-labeled antigen, also called tracer, bound to the antibodies will decrease as the concentration of unlabeled antigen from the sample increases. This can be measured after separating antibody-bound from free tracer and counting one or the other, or both fractions (Skelly et al. 1973, Goldsmith 1975, Davies 2013). However, due to health concerns regarding working processes with radioactive materials, the use of RIA has been reduced as much as possible in recent times (Lequin 2005) and currently requires specific laboratory standards and authorization. Thereby, the RIA method has been nearly replaced by enzyme immunoassays (EIA) (Aydin 2015). In this technique, the radioactive isotopes were replaced by enzyme-labeled markers. The main advantages of EIA are the reduced health danger issues due to the non-existence of radioactivity with concurrent high specificity (Kunkel 1991). Based on the technique, EIAs can also be differentiated into competitive and non-competitive assays and homogenous and heterogenous assays (Davies 2013). In homogenous assays, the amount of product produced depends on the extent of immune complex reaction. The activity of the enzyme is changed by binding the enzyme-labelled ligand to the antibody and both reactions can take place concurrently in the same solution (Engvall and Perlmann 1971, Engvall 2010, Davies 2013, Weeks et al. 2013). By contrast, the enzymatic activity is not coupled with the immune reaction in heterogeneous assays. Thus, the bound and free reactants must be separated by a washing step, also called bound-free separation (Davies 2013). The advantages of this technique are the broad range of molecule sizes which can be measured and the removal of potentially interfering substances from the matrix before the start of the quantification step and, thereby, increasing the sensitivity of the assay (Engvall and Perlmann 1971, Engvall 2010, Aydin 2015). The most well-known heterogeneous EIA is probably the enzyme-linked immunosorbent assay (ELISA) (Engvall and Perlmann 1971). Enzymes in ELISA are, for example, alkaline phosphatase or horseradish peroxidase, used to convert a substrate which is most often a chromogen, a normally colorless molecule, into a colored end product (Weeks et al. 2013, Aydin 2015). Thus, the color intensity of the end product is measured as absorbance in optical density with a spectrophotometer (Weeks et al. 2013). The measued absorbance measured directly and proportionally reflects the amount of the enzyme converted substrate and is directly proportional to the amount of antigen captured (Engvall and Perlmann 1971, Engvall 2010, Aydin 2015).

Another frequently used EIA technique is based on chemiluminescence and the detection of light emitted by a chemical reaction (Weeks et al. 2013). The simple colorimetric detection method in these chemiluminescence immunoassays (CLIA) is changed to detection luminescence (Dudley 1990, Kricka 1991). Based on an initiated chemical reaction, one of the reaction products yielded in an electronically excited state produces light on falling to the ground state (Jandreski 1998). Luminol, acridinium esters, peroxyoxalates, dioxetanes or tris(2,2'bipyridyl)ruthenium(II) can be used as chemiluminescent labels (Weeks et al. 2013). Whereas luminol and other derivates need a catalyzer for the reaction, firstly, complicating the procedure and, secondly, potentially impairing the further light-emitting reaction, reagents such as acridinium esters do not need catalyzers and, thereby, accelerate the process.

Therefore, acridinium esters are most often used in CLIAs (Weeks et al. 2013). The sensitivity of CLIAs is appreciably higher compared to other methods measuring optical density (Kricka 1991, Jandreski 1998, Wild 2013) and, in contrast to, for example, reagents from RIA, most chemiluminescent reagents and conjugates are stable for long periods. Furthermore, there are no health concerns reported for the chemiluminescent reagents (Kricka 1991). Additional benefits from economical points of views are the relatively low amounts of reagents required compared to other EIA methods and, therefore, the reduced costs. Moreover, most of the CLIA systems are widely available and many of them run on automated platforms, which further simplifies operations in routine diagnostic laboratories. Currently, all the methods described have been used to quantify insulin in human and animal specimens. However, CLIA analyses are probably used most frequently based on their relative advantages compared to the other methods. In addition to analysis using immunoassay methods, insulin can also be quantified by utilizing liquid chromatography and high-resolution/high-accuracy mass spectrometry (LC-MS), which is often considered to be the gold standard for quantification. Several studies using LC-MS reported a convincing accuracy and analytical sensitivity in the detection of insulin (Chen et al. 2013; Van Der Gugten et al. 2016).

2.4 QUANTIFICATION OF EQUINE INSULIN BASED ON IMMUNOASSAYS

Most immunoassays used in veterinary medicine for analyzing insulin concentrations in equine serum or plasma samples were originally designed for human diagnostics and research. In contrast to most laboratory species, specific immunoassays for the quantification of equine insulin based on antibodies directed against epitopes of the equine insulin are not commercially available. Nevertheless, multiple assays have been released and advertised to be species-specific.

Initially, a human-specific RIA (Coat-a-Count Insulin RIA, Siemens Medical Solutions) has been intensively validated for use in horses (Freestone et al. 1991; Tinworth et al. 2009) and was used frequently in several research studies (Eiler et al. 2005;

Frank et al. 2006) and in clinical settings and for diagnostic purposes in veterinary laboratories.

Several studies have been performed since to evaluate different commercially available immunoassays for the quantification of equine insulin (Öberg et al. 2011; Tinworth et al. 2011; Borer-Weir et al. 2012; Banse et al. 2014; Carslake et al. 2017). Striking differences in the insulin concentrations measured have been detected when various assays were compared. Banse et al. (2014) compared the previously well validated human-specific RIA (Coat-a-Count Insulin RIA, Siemens Medical Solutions) with a commercially available human-specific CLIA (IMMULITE 1000, Siemens Medical Solutions) for the measurement of equine insulin and reported that both methods had poor concordance. By contrast, Carslake et al. (2017) defined a CLIA (IMMULITE 2000, Siemens Medical Solutions) as a highly repeatable assay which is suitable for within and between horse comparisons in a retrospective study comparing results supplied by the new assay with the old RIA data (Coat-a-Count Insulin RIA, Siemens Medical Solutions). However, the authors mentioned that at concentrations commonly used for the diagnosis of ID ($\leq$ 100 µIU/mL), results from the CLIA (IMMULITE 2000, Siemens Medical Solutions) tended to be lower than from the previously well validated human-specific RIA (Coat-a-Count Insulin RIA, Siemens Medical Solutions). Furthermore, Tinworth (2011) found missing concordance between methods when comparing six commercially available assays used for quantifying equine insulin. Out of the six assays investigated, only two performed satisfactorily: The human-specific RIA already mentioned previously (Coat-a-Count Insulin RIA, Siemens Medical Solutions) and the equine-optimized porcine-specific ELISA (Equine insulin ELISA, Mercodia AB). However, the RIA only performed satisfactorily after modification of the dilution procedure by using a charcoal-stripped equine plasma instead of the assay buffer provided by the manufacturer. Nevertheless, they reported missing accordance and weak correlations for the two immunoassays relative to the LC-MS measurements. It should be noted that the LC-MS techniques used required specific sample preparation with previous antibody-antigen binding processes which might have impaired the results and the technology (Tinworth et al. 2011). Similar to human medicine, the LC-MS technology has previously been used in equid, although to analyze equine urine and plasma samples for insulin in the context of doping issues instead of routine clinical diagnostics (Ho et al. 2008, 2011). Borer-Weir et al. (2012) reported a good agreement between the human-specific RIA (Coat-a-Count Insulin RIA, Siemens Medical Solutions) and equine-optimized porcine-specific ELISA (Equine Insulin ELISA, Mercodia AB) for samples containing concentrations of less than 175 µIU/mL but further highlighted important complications and missing accordance when high insulin concentrations measured in samples were evaluated and compared.

2.5 CLINICAL STANDARDS AND VALIDATION OF IMMUNOASSAYS IN VETERINARY CLINICAL PATHOLOGY

The accuracy of laboratory methods is crucial to ensure safe and reliable diagnostic procedures based on clinical pathology parameters (American Society for Clinical Veterinary Pathology 2009, U.S. Department of Health and Human Services, Food and Drug Administration 2018). Minor test variability is highly consequential because inaccurate test results with subtle differences in parameter concentration levels might indicate clinically important disease-mediated changes. However, hormones are present in very low concentrations (10^{-11} to 10^{-9} M) in contrast to other routinely determined clinical chemistry parameters that are generally present at much higher concentrations (10^{-5} to 10^{-3} M). Therefore, laboratory analyses of hormones can generally be challenging (Haddad et al. 2019) and often requires more complex and, based on the low concentrations, very sensitive analytical methods compared to clinical chemistry analyses. In 2009, the American Society for Clinical Veterinary Pathology (ASCVP) published guidelines and recommendations for appropriate assay validation used for veterinary medicine. These guidelines focus on the assessment of accuracy, linearity, analytical range, precision, lower limit of detection (LLOD) and functional sensitivity (American Society for Clinical Veterinary Pathology 2009). Accuracy and determination of analytical range are defined based on linearity (Lee et al. 2006, Andreasson et al. 2015, U.S. Department of Health and Human Services, Food and Drug Administration 2018). Accuracy describes the relationship of the average measured value to the true value (Lee et al. 2006, U.S. Department of

Health and Human Services, Food and Drug Administration 2018). The difference between both is stated as bias and may be proportional if the assay reads a constant percentage higher or lower than the true value or constant if the assay reads a constant concentration higher or lower than the true value (American Society for Clinical Veterinary Pathology 2009, U.S. Department of Health and Human Services, Food and Drug Administration 2018). The linearity is defined as the proportional signal between the analyte concentration and the signal detected (Christenson and Duh 2012, Lee et al. 2006). This linearity should be assessed from low to high analyte concentrations and in serial dilution steps to prove consistent performance. This allows the detection of LLOD and upper limit of detection, representing concentration limits, which require further sample preparation as dilutions (U.S. Department of Health and Human Services, Food and Drug Administration 2018). The sensitivity is defined as the lowest measurable concentration of the analyte that can still be safely differentiated from the blank (International Organization for Standardization 1994). The LLOD describes the analytical sensitivity and is calculated as the mean of the blank or zero calibrator plus two or three standard deviations and crucial for describing an assay's performance (International Organization for Standardization 1994, Lee et al. 2006). Values close to the calculated limits are not particularly reliable. In contrast to the analytical sensitivity, the functional sensitivity of the assay is calculated as the lowest concentration for which the coefficient of variation (CV) is less than 20 % (Davies 2013) or the mean of the lowest spiked sample with a CV less than 20 % (American Society for Clinical Veterinary Pathology 2009). To cover the range of clinically relevant concentrations, the assay's analytical range should be appropriate and at least six standards for calculation of an appropriate standard curve are recommended (Valentin et al. 2011). Selectivity of the assay can be checked by the measurement of recovery (Lee et al. 2006, U.S. Department of Health and Human Services, Food and Drug Administration 2018). Therefore, the measured increase in concentration is divided by the predicted increase in concentration and multiplied by 100. Recovery should be assessed in samples containing high analyte concentrations (U.S. Department of Health and Human Services, Food and Drug Administration 2018). If not available, the samples can be spiked with a standard in order to cover a broader range of the concentration. However, in this case, the samples dilution should not exceed 10 % to avoid impaired sample matrix. The concentration of the analyte should cover the clinically relevant concentration range for recovery studies (American Society for Clinical Veterinary Pathology 2009). Clinical practice samples containing high concentrations of the analyte may require dilution if the analytical range of the assay does not fit properly. This is especially important in terms of analyses from samples with marked differences between the basal or resting concentrations and analyte concentrations provoked under stimulated or inhibited conditions. Therefore, dilution of samples is often necessary and a common issue. The recovery upon dilution can be estimated to detect potential interference with the dilution procedure (Lee et al. 2006). The dilution of the sample should lie parallel to the calibration curve and parallelism should be checked across the working range of the assay (Lee et al. 2006, Davies 2013, U.S. Department of Health and Human Services, Food and Drug Administration 2018). However, dilution of samples can be challenging if the dilution medium does not fit with the sample matrix. In these cases, charcoal-stripped serum or plasma can improve assay performance with diluted samples (American Society for Clinical Veterinary Pathology 2009). The assay precision describes the repeatability of an analytical technique and can be calculated as imprecision, an estimate of the error in an analytical technique (International Organization for Standardization 1994, Andreasson et al. 2015). Imprecision can be defined by the calculation of the CV and, thereby, reflects the random error (Findlay et al. 2000). The standard deviation of all measures is divided by the mean and multiplied by 100 to calculate the CV (Jensen and Kjelgaard-Hansen 2006). Within-run precision describes variations within a single run of the assay and is calculated as intra-assay CV. The intra-assay CV should be calculated on 20 replicates of one sample within a single run of the assay. The CV normally increases with very low or very high analyte concentrations (Davies 2013). Therefore, replicates of at least three samples covering the analytical range of the assay should be performed. Between-run precision is based on the calculation of inter-assay CVs. Therefore, the same sample should be measured on different runs of the assay. The intra- and inter-assay CV should not generally exceed 25 % (Valentin et al. 2011). Despite many other assay-specific characteristics, the antibody specificity is essential for an appropriate performance. The assay specificity describes the ability of an antibody to produce a measurable response only for the analyte of interest (International Organization for Standardization 1994, U.S. Department of Health and Human Services, Food and Drug Administration 2018, Davies 2013). Samples can be spiked with proteins with a similar structure to the targeted analyte and checked for recovery and, thereby, assess cross-reactivity to test specificity. However, it is important to consider that cross-reactivity may vary across the assay range. An assay's antibody specificity might be different based on the usage of polyclonal, monoclonal or recombinant antibodies (Davies 2013, Liddell 2013). Furthermore, specificity should be assessed in clinical concentration ranges and on supraphysiological levels. Recovery is generally considered to be adequate if accuracy is 70–130 % compared to unspiked samples and CV is < 25 % (Valentin et al. 2011). Furthermore, the assay should be tested for potential interference or matrix effects caused by other components of the sample except the specific analyte to be quantified (American Society for Clinical Veterinary Pathology 2009, U.S. Department of Health and Human Services, Food and Drug Administration 2018). Several substances, such as bilirubin, hemoglobin or lipids, can interfere with assay performance and impair results (Dimeski 2008).

Comparison among assays or especially comparison of a new method against a previously established method can be challenging. It is recommended to use at least 40 samples, covering the working range of the assay (American Society for Clinical Veterinary Pathology 2009). Mathematical and statistical evaluation and comparison should include Bland-Altman analyses as well as correlation and regression analyses. However, correlation analyses only test whether the two methods are associated and do not describe the degree of agreement. In principle, low correlations can be improved by increasing the sample size but indicate discrepancies between the assays investigated and preclude interchangeable use of both (Stockl et al. 1998). If correlation analyses are sufficient, further regression analysis provides additional information. Least square or Deming regression analyses may provide more reliable information than simple correlation or linear regression. They can be used to determine whether constant or proportional systematic errors occur. Proportional error is interpreted by the slope and is indicated by a slope ≠1. By contrast, constant error is indicated by the intercept ≠1 (Stockl et al. 1998). Significant systematic errors preclude the interchangeable usage of both assays and may complicate clinical usage. Particularly from a clinician's point of view, diagnostic consequences such as the discordance of analyte concentrations with previously defined references ranges due to a disagreement of assays can be challenging (Haeckel and Wosniok 2004).

3 SCOPE OF THE THESIS – HYPOTHESIS AND AIMS

The objective of this research project was firstly to evaluate quantification of equine insulin under consideration of clinical demands and conditions and secondly to optimize assessment of equine ID and IR by a combination of appropriate dynamic diagnostic testing and quantification of equine insulin with reliable immunoassay methods.

Hypotheses:

1. Equine insulin concentrations measured with different immunoassays will differ significantly.

2. Dynamic diagnostic testing with OGT and analysis of blood samples with an appropriate immunoassay provides reliable assessment of equine ID.

3. Selection of immunoassay influences results and interpretation of OGT and CGIT.

The aims of the study:

1. The first aim of this study was to re-validate an equine-optimized insulin ELISA.

2. The second aim of the study was to compare three immunoassays frequently used for the analyses of equine insulin and to test their clinical applicability in assessing ID in basal blood samples and blood samples obtained during standard dosed OGT via naso-gastric tubing.

3. The third aim of the study was to describe variations in insulin responses to standard dosed OGT via naso-gastric tubing and to provide a clinical useful cut-off value for ID when using the insulin quantification with the equine-optimized insulin ELISA.

4. The fourth aim of the study was to compare two frequently used immunoassays for the analyses of endogenous equine insulin or exogenous non-equine insulin in two large cohorts of blood samples obtained from OGT to diagnose ID and from CGIT procedure to diagnose tissue IR.

4 MATERIALS AND METHODS

4.1 ANIMALS AND SAMPLES

4.1.1 PART I

In the first part of the study, 40 blood samples from seventeen horses and ponies were used for comparison of immunoassays. Horses and ponies were of different breeds. The mean age was 14 ± 6 years and the mean weight 478 ± 179 kg. Samples were collected under basal fasted conditions as well as stimulated conditions during OGT with provoked hyperinsulinemia. Blood samples were collected via jugular vein catheter (EquiCath[TM] Fastflow, Braun Vet Care GmbH, Tuttlingen, Germany or Intraflon 12 G, Vygon SA, Ecouen, France), transferred into plain tubes for serum preparation (Vacuette[®] Greiner Bio One, Frickenhausen, Germany) and were incubated at room temperature for 60 min, centrifuged at 3000 x g for 6 min and serum was stored at −80 °C. Prior to analyses samples were thawed once and split into different aliquots and were re-frozen until analysis (see 5 Manuscript I, Methods, Animals and Samples, page 35).

4.1.2 PART II

In the second part of the study, blood samples from 56 horses and ponies were used for analyses of insulin responses after glycemic challenge during OGT procedure. Included horses and ponies were 23 warmblood horses, 19 Icelandic horses, 5 Shetland ponies and 9 ponies of various breeds. There were 26 mares, 25 geldings and 5 stallions with a mean age of 15 ± 6 years and mean weight of 473 ± 136 kg. Blood samples were collected via jugular vein catheter (EquiCath[TM] Fastflow, Braun Vet Care GmbH, Tuttlingen, Germany or Intraflon 12 G, Vygon SA, Ecouen, France), transferred into plain tubes for serum preparation (Vacuette[®] Greiner Bio One, Frickenhausen, Germany), incubated at room temperature for 60 min, centrifuged at 1000 x g for 6 min, were aliquoted and stored at − 80 °C until further analysis (see 6. Manuscript II, page 48).

25

4.1.3 PART III

In the third part of the study, 268 blood samples obtained during PO glycemic challenge performed by OGT and during IV challenge test performed by CGIT have been collcted from nine healthy warmblood breed horses. There were five mares, two geldings and two stallions. The mean age was 16±7.8 years and the mean weight 539±68 kg. Blood samples were collected via jugular vein catheter (EquiCath[TM] Fastflow, Braun Vet Care GmbH, Tuttlingen, Germany or Intraflon 12 G, Vygon SA, Ecouen, France), placed into plain tubes for serum preparation (Vacuette[®] Greiner Bio One, Frickenhausen, Germany), incubated at room temperature for 60 min, centrifuged at 1000 x g for 6 min, were aliquoted and stored at 80°C until further analysis (see 7. Manuscript III, page 56–57).

4.2 IMMUNOASSAYS

4.2.1 RADIOIMMUNOASSAY (RIA)

Sample analyses by RIA were performed using a porcine-specific insulin RIA (Porcine Insulin RIA, Millipore, St. Charles, MO, USA) (see 5 Manuscript I, Methods, Assays, page 35–36).

4.2.2 IMMUNORADIOMETRIC ASSAY (IRMA)

Sample analyses by IRMA were performed using a human-specific IRMA (Insulin(e) IRMA KIT, Beckman Coulter, Prague, Czech Republic). (see 7 Manuscript III, Materials and Methods, Insulin analyses, page 57–58).

4.2.3 ENZYME-LINKED IMMUNOSORBENT ASSAY (ELISA)

Sample analyses by ELISA were performed using an equine-optimized porcine-specific insulin ELISA (Equine Insulin ELISA, Mercodia AB, Uppsala, Sweden) (see 5 Manuscript I, Methods, Assays, page 35–36 and 7 Manuscript III, Materials and Methods, Insulin analyses, page 57–58).

26

4.2.4 CHEMILUMINESCENCE IMMUNOASSAY (CLIA)

Sample analyses by CLIA were performed using a human-specific insulin CLIA (ADVIA Centaur XP Insulin Assay, Siemens Healthcare Diagnostics GmbH, Eschborn, Germany) (see 5 Manuscript I, Methods, Assays, page 35–36).

4.3 DIAGNOSTIC TESTS FOR ASSESSMENT OF ID AND IR

4.3.1 ORAL GLUCOSE TEST (OGT)

For implementation of OGT 1 g/kg BW glucose powder (Glukose, WDT, Garbsen, Germany) dissolved in two liters water was administered by naso-gastric tubing. Blood samples were collected via jugular vein catheter (EquiCath^{TM} Fastflow, Braun Vet Care GmbH, Germany or Intraflon 12 G, Vygon SA, Ecouen, France) (see 5 Manuscript I, Methods, Animals and samples, page 35; 6 Manuscript II, page 48; 7 Manuscript III, Materials and Methods, Animals and Samples, page 57–58)

4.3.2 COMBINED INSULIN GLUCOSE TEST (CGIT)

For implementation of the CGIT two intravenous indwelling catheters (EquiCath^{TM} Fastflow, Braun Vet Care GmbH, Germany) were aseptically implanted in each jugular vein of the horses. One catheter was used for administration of glucose solution and insulin, whereas the second one was used for the collection of blood samples for three hours. The CGIT was performed by IV injection of 150 mg/kg BW glucose solution (Glucose 500 mg/mL, B. Braun Melsungen AG, Germany) within 1 minute, immediately followed by injection of 0.1 IU/kg BW porcine zinc-insulin (Caninsulin® 40 I.E./ml, MSD, Unterschleißheim, Germany) and 20 mL saline solution (NaCl; 0,9 %; B. Braun Melsungen AG, Germany) to flush the catheter. (see 7 Manuscript III, Materials and Methods, Animals and Samples, page 56–57)

4.4 STATISTICS

4.4.1 PART I

Statistical analysis was performed using GraphPad Prism software (GraphPad Prism, Version 6.02 for Windows, GraphPad Inc. La Jolla, CA, USA). The Shapiro-Wilk normality test was used to assess the normality of data distribution. Wilcoxon matchedpairs signed rank test, Spearman correlation and Deming regression analyses were used to compare results from different assays and to verify relationships between the three methods. Bland-Altman analysis was performed to calculate method-dependent bias and limits of agreements. Wilcoxon matched-pairs signed rank test was also used to examine the effect of repeated freezing and thawing on the stability of equine insulin. Statistical significance was set at p < 0.05. (see 5 Manuscript I, Methods, Statistics and calculations, page 36–37).

4.4.2 PART II

Statistical analysis was performed in R 3.4.0.6 (R version 3.4.0, The R Foundation for Statistical Computing). Data analysis was performed using a model based clustering method provided by the mclust R-package in combination with a scaled singular value decomposition (SVD) projection for improved initialization. Two clusters retained by the mclust algorithm with improved initialization relate to another. The separation line between the two clusters at 120 min was at 105 µIU/mL insulin. The pseudomedian with 95% confidence interval for both clusters as estimated from the Hodges-Lehmann estimator. For calculation of the cut-off value the 97.5% quantile of the cluster 1 was used (see 6 Manuscript II, page 48–49).

4.4.3 PART III

Data analysis and statistics were performed using GraphPad Prism software (version 7.02; GraphPad Inc. La Jolla, CA, USA). Data was tested for normality using Shapiro-Wilk normality test. Wilcoxon signed rank test, Spearman correlation and Deming regression analyses were used to compare results from different assays to evaluate relationships between the both methods. Bland-Altman analysis was performed to calculate method-dependent bias and 95 % limits of agreement between both methods. Repeated measures two-way ANOVA with Sidak´s multiple comparisons test was performed to compare results supplied by RIA and ELISA in OGT and CGIT over the testing period. Statistical significance was accepted when p<0.05 (see 7 Manuscript III, Materials and Methods, Data analyses and Statistics, page 58).

5 PART I – MANUSCRIPT I

Comparison of three different methods for quantification of equine insulin

Tobias Warnken[1+2*], Korinna Huber[3], Karsten Feige[1]

[1]   Clinic for Horses, University of Veterinary Medicine Hannover, Foundation, Bünteweg 9, 30559 Hannover, Germany

[2]   Department of Physiology, University of Veterinary Medicine Hannover, Foundation, Bischofsholer Damm 15, 30173 Hannover, Germany

[3]   Institute of Animal Science, Faculty of Agricultural Sciences, University of Hohenheim, Fruwirthstraße 35, 70599 Stuttgart, Germany

*Corresponding author: Tobias Warnken

BMC Veterinary Research 2016; 12(1): 196.

Accepted: 1st September 2016; available online: 9th September 2016.

DOI: 10.1186/s12917-016-0828-z

https://bmcvetres.biomedcentral.com/articles/10.1186/s12917-016-0828-z

Contribution to the manuscript

TW, KH and KF designed the study. TW collected and analyzed data, wrote

the manuscript and made figures. KH and KF helped to edit the manuscript.

All authors read and approved the final manuscript.

Abstract

Background: Exact analysis of equine insulin in blood samples is the key element for assessing insulin resistance or insulin dysregulation in horses. However, previous studies indicated marked differences in insulin concentrations obtained from sample analyses with different immunoassays. Most assays used in veterinary medicine are originally designed for use in human diagnostics and are based on antibodies directed against human insulin, although amino acid sequences between equine and human insulin differ. Species-specific assays are being used more frequently and seem to provide advantages compared to human-specific assays. The aim of this study was to compare three immunoassays, one porcine-specific insulin enzymelinked immunosorbent assay (ELISA), advertised to be specific for equine insulin, one porcine-specific insulin radioimmunoassay (RIA) and one human-specific insulin chemiluminescence immunoassay (CLIA), all three widely used in veterinary laboratories for the analysis of equine insulin. Furthermore, we tested their clinical applicability in assessing insulin resistance and dysregulation by analysis of basal blood and blood samples obtained during a dynamic diagnostic stimulation test (OGT) with elevated insulin concentrations.

Results: Insulin values obtained from the ELISA, RIA and CLIA, investigated for analyses of basal blood samples differed significantly between all three assays. Analyses of samples obtained during dynamic diagnostic stimulation testing with consecutively higher insulin concentrations revealed significantly ($p < 0.001$) lower insulin concentrations supplied by the CLIA compared to the ELISA. However, values measured by ELISA were intermediate and not different to those measured by RIA. Calculated recovery upon dilution, as a marker for assay accuracy in diluted samples, was 98 ± 4 % for ELISA, 160 ± 41 % for RIA and 101 ± 11 % for CLIA.

Conclusions: Our results indicate that insulin concentrations of one sample measured by different methods vary greatly and should be interpreted carefully. Consideration of the immunoassay method and reliable assay-specific reference ranges are of particular importance especially in clinical cases where small changes in insulin levels can cause false classification in terms of insulin sensitivity of horses and ponies.

Keywords: Horse, Equine, Insulin, Quantification, ELISA, RIA, CLIA, EMS

Warnken *et al. BMC Veterinary Research* (2016) 12:196
DOI 10.1186/s12917-016-0828-z

BMC Veterinary Research

Comparison of three different methods for the quantification of equine insulin

CrossMark

T. Warnken[1,3*], K. Huber[2] and K. Feige[3]

Abstract

Background: Exact analysis of equine insulin in blood samples is the key element for assessing insulin resistance or insulin dysregulation in horses. However, previous studies indicated marked differences in insulin concentrations obtained from sample analyses with different immunoassays. Most assays used in veterinary medicine are originally designed for use in human diagnostics and are based on antibodies directed against human insulin, although amino acid sequences between equine and human insulin differ. Species-specific assays are being used more frequently and seem to provide advantages compared to human-specific assays. The aim of this study was to compare three immunoassays, one porcine-specific insulin enzyme-linked immunosorbent assay (ELISA), advertised to be specific for equine insulin, one porcine-specific insulin radioimmunoassay (RIA) and one human-specific insulin chemiluminescence immunoassay (CLIA), all three widely used in veterinary laboratories for the analysis of equine insulin. Furthermore, we tested their clinical applicability in assessing insulin resistance and dysregulation by analysis of basal blood and blood samples obtained during a dynamic diagnostic stimulation test (OGT) with elevated insulin concentrations.

Results: Insulin values obtained from the ELISA, RIA and CLIA, investigated for analyses of basal blood samples differed significantly between all three assays. Analyses of samples obtained during dynamic diagnostic stimulation testing with consecutively higher insulin concentrations revealed significantly ($p < 0.001$) lower insulin concentrations supplied by the CLIA compared to the ELISA. However, values measured by ELISA were intermediate and not different to those measured by RIA. Calculated recovery upon dilution, as a marker for assay accuracy in diluted samples, was 98 ± 4 % for ELISA, 160 ± 41 % for RIA and 101 ± 11 % for CLIA.

Conclusions: Our results indicate that insulin concentrations of one sample measured by different methods vary greatly and should be interpreted carefully. Consideration of the immunoassay method and reliable assay-specific reference ranges are of particular importance especially in clinical cases where small changes in insulin levels can cause false classification in terms of insulin sensitivity of horses and ponies.

Keywords: Horse, Equine, Insulin, Quantification, ELISA, RIA, CLIA, EMS

* Correspondence: tobias.warnken@tiho-hannover.de
[1]Department of Physiology, University of Veterinary Medicine Hannover,
Foundation, Bischofsholer Damm 15, 30173 Hannover, Germany
[3]Clinic for Horses, University of Veterinary Medicine Hannover, Foundation,
Bünteweg 9, 30559 Hannover, Germany
Full list of author information is available at the end of the article

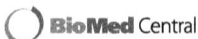

MANUSCRIPT I

Warnken et al. BMC Veterinary Research (2016) 12:196

Page 2 of 10

Background

The equine metabolic syndrome (EMS) has attracted increasing attention in equine veterinary practice in recent years and is becoming more common due to today's horse husbandry and feeding practices. Different diagnostic tests to determine dysregulation of glucose and insulin homeostasis in horses are currently used to diagnose EMS. Tests are based on quantitative measures either of basal serum insulin concentration in fasted and non-fasted horses or of increased insulin concentration stimulated by oral [1, 2] or intravenous [3] dynamic diagnostic tests. Complex hyperinsulinaemic euglycaemic clamp (HEC) tests, which were considered to be the gold standard for assessment of insulin resistance (IR) [4], were usually reserved to research approaches due to their complex and expensive implementation. High insulin indicative of IR or insulin dysregulation (ID) in EMS horses is one of the features associated with this metabolic disorder [5]. Exact pathophysiology resulting in IR is not known to date. Several hypothesis leading to the clinical signs have been discussed in literature. Increased insulin degradation or neutralization, decreased binding of insulin to its receptor, as well as impaired downstream signaling were described. Whereas the term IR used in context with EMS is mainly characterized by reduced tissue response of insulin-dependent tissues the newly introduced term ID is used to describe in summary abnormalities of insulin metabolism [5]. Therefore, an exact quantification of insulin by laboratory analysis is the most important and challenging step to diagnose EMS-related changes in insulin regulation. Several immunoassay methods for the quantification of insulin in equine serum or plasma samples are commercially available. However, due to the use of different methods for quantifying equine insulin, discrepancies between results obtained from different studies have occurred [6, 7]. Since no assay with a specific antibody against equine insulin is available, most of the commercial immunoassays are based on antibodies directed against human or non-equine insulin. Only one enzyme-linked immunosorbent assay (ELISA) advertised by the manufacturer as being specific for measuring equine insulin is commercially available[1], and this is based on anti-porcine insulin antibodies. This assay has been validated for use in horses [8] and has already been used successfully in several studies [9, 10].

The aim of our study was to compare the results of this equine-optimized porcine-specific ELISA with results obtained from a radioimmunoassay[2] (RIA) and a chemiluminescence immunoassay[3] (CLIA) for measurements of equine insulin in serum samples. Furthermore, the second aim of the study was to evaluate the applicability of the three assays for samples obtained from horses and ponies under fasted conditions and

from horses and ponies with stimulated insulin secretion during diagnostic procedure.

Methods

Animals and samples

Forty blood serum samples were collected from seventeen horses and ponies of different breeds, age (14 ± 6 years), weight (478 ± 179 kg) and body condition score (6.8 ± 1.1) to obtain samples with a broad range of insulin concentrations. Blood samples from healthy, university-owned horses were collected during a study, which has been approved by the ethics committee within the University of Veterinary Medicine, Hannover, and the State Office for Consumer Protection and Food Safety in accordance with the German Animal Welfare Law (LAVES–Reference number: 33.14 42502-04-13/1259). Blood samples from insulin dysregulated horses and ponies were collected during routine diagnostic procedures in the Clinic for Horses and informed consent was obtained from the clients for publication. Blood samples were collected after fasting the horses overnight (basal, $n = 20$), and additionally after stimulation by an oral glucose testing (OGT, $n = 20$) procedure [2]. OGT was carried out by administering 1 g/kg btw glucose powder dissolved in two liters water by naso-gastrical-tubation. Samples were collected via jugular vein catheter, transferred into plain tubes[4] for serum preparation and were incubated at room temperature for 1 h, centrifuged at 3000 g for 6 min and serum was stored at –80 °C. Prior to analyses samples were thawed once and split into different aliquots containing the required volume for each assay. Afterwards, they were re-frozen and sent on dry ice to the laboratories.

Assays

The porcine-specific insulin assay[1] is a solid phase two-side sandwich ELISA optimized for the quantification of equine insulin in serum or plasma. It is based on monoclonal mouse anti-porcine insulin antibodies coupled to plate and free monoclonal mouse anti-porcine insulin antibody conjugate labeled with horseradish peroxidase. Porcine insulin is used for calibrators to compute calibration curve via cubic spline regression. The limit of detection for this assay is 1.17 µIU/mL, but concentrations of samples with absorbance below the lowest calibrator (2.34 µIU/mL) should not be calculated. Cross reactivity of the assay is stated at 100 % for porcine insulin and 22 % with human insulin (according to the manufacturer's protocol) (Table 1).

For sample analysis by RIA, a porcine-specific one-site insulin RIA[2] was used. This assay is based on ^{125}I-labeled insulin and used guinea pig anti-porcine insulin antibodies and goat anti-guinea pig IgG antibodies. Purified human recombinant insulin preparations were used as standards

Warnken *et al. BMC Veterinary Research* (2016) 12:196

Table 1 Information about the three assays examined for quantification of equine insulin

Assay	Standards	Primary antibody	Second antibody
Mercodia Equine Insulin ELISA	Porcine insulin	Mouse monoclonal anti-porcine insulin	Mouse monoclonal anti-porcine insulin HRP-conjugate
Millipore Porcine Insulin RIA	Human recombinant insulin	Guinea pig anti-porcine insulin	Goat anti-guinea pig IgG
Siemens ADVIA Centaur Insulin Assay	-[a]	Monoclonal mouse anti-insulin AE-conjugate	Monoclonal mouse anti-insulin coupled to paramagnetic particles

[a]No information available

for calibration. The manufacturer's protocol referred to the assay's limit of linearity of 200 μIU/mL and recommended diluting the samples which have greater concentrations with the assay buffer. The limit of detection for this assay is 1.61 μIU/mL when 100 μl of sample is used. The cross-reactivity of the assay is stated at 100 % for porcine insulin, 100 % for human insulin and 90 % for bovine insulin. No information about cross-reactivity for equine insulin is given by the manufacturer. Measurements with the RIA were performed by a commercial veterinary endocrinology laboratory.

A human-specific insulin chemiluminescent immuno-assay[4] with two-site sandwich technique and direct chemiluminescent technology was used for the sample analysis by CLIA. The assay is based on monoclonal mouse anti-insulin antibodies and chemiluminescent detection with monoclonal mouse anti-insulin antibodies labeled with acridinium ester. The limit of detection of this assay is 0.5 μIU/mL and the measuring range is from 1.0 to 300 μIU/mL. No information about cross-reactivity for equine insulin is given by the manufacturer. Measurements using the CLIA were performed by a commercial veterinary laboratory. Due to the fact that all tested assays use no equine standards, all the assays only provide an approximation of equine insulin concentrations.

Revalidation of the equine-optimized porcine-specific insulin ELISA

Intra-assay CV was calculated by division of the standard deviation by the corresponding mean of 15 replicates of equine serum samples with low (mean: 2.34 μIU/mL) and medium (mean: 108.81 μIU/mL) insulin concentrations. Inter-assay CV was calculated by division of the standard deviation by the corresponding mean of replicate samples, each measured on 25 different plates. Commercial controls[5] with low (5.03 μIU/mL), medium (18.84 μIU/mL) and high (60.84 μIU/mL) insulin concentrations (classifications according to manufacturer), and equine serum samples with low (mean: 10.53 μIU/mL) and medium (mean: 109.98 μIU/mL) insulin concentrations were used for the calculation of concentration-dependent inter-assay CVs. The recovery upon dilution (RUD) and the linearity of dilution were calculated to prove accuracy. A sample selected with a medium insulin concentration (99.45 μIU/mL) was measurable without any dilution and

in five different dilution steps up to the 1:40 ratio dilution within the calibration range of the assay. Sample buffer[6] was used for dilution and at least 40 μl of the equine serum sample.

Comparison of methods

Basal serum samples and simulated samples from the OGT procedure were measured undiluted in all three assays for comparison of methods. Moreover, stimulated samples were additionally measured diluted in a ratio of 1:4 with sample buffer[6] to calculate the RUD for each assay to prove accuracy in the measurement of dilution procedure. The RUD was calculated as a percentage recovery of the insulin concentration in the diluted sample related to the corresponding undiluted samples. The RUD analyses were performed without the knowledge of the laboratories commissioned.

Stability of insulin after freezing, thawing and eight weeks of storage

In order to investigate the effect of repeated freezing and thawing on the stability of insulin in serum samples measured by equine-optimized, porcine-specific ELISA, 33 samples were thawed, measured and refrozen at −80 °C. Eight weeks later, samples were thawed at ambient temperature for 1 h and measured again. Samples covering a broad range of insulin concentrations were chosen to match the assay's analytical range from 2.34 to 175.5 μIU/mL. The samples were subdivided into three subgroups of low (3.51–15.21 μIU/mL), medium (30.42–90.09 μIU/mL) and high (92.43–125.19 μIU/mL) concentrations with eleven samples in each subgroup.

Statistics and calculations

Data analysis was performed using GraphPad Prism software[7]. The Shapiro-Wilk normality test was used to assess the normality of data distribution. Wilcoxon matched-pairs signed rank test, Spearman correlation and Deming regression analyses were used to compare results from different assays and to verify relationships between the three methods. In cases of assay-based non-detectable insulin concentrations, the corresponding samples were excluded from the statistics. Bland-Altman analysis was performed to calculate method-dependent bias and limits of agreements. Wilcoxon matched-pairs signed rank test was also

MANUSCRIPT I

Warnken et al. BMC Veterinary Research (2016) 12:196   Page 4 of 10

used to examine the effect of repeated freezing and thawing on the stability of equine insulin. Statistical significance was set at $p < 0.05$.

Results

In re-validation experiments, intra-assay CV was 4.61 % at low insulin concentrations (2.34 µIU/mL) and 1.91 % at medium insulin concentrations (108.81 µIU/mL) using the equine-specific insulin ELISA. The inter-assay CV was 5.27 %, 3.24 % and 3.17 % for the low (reference value 5.03 µIU/mL insulin), medium (reference value 18.84 µIU/mL insulin) and high (reference value 60.84 µIU/mL insulin) commercial controls, respectively. Inter-assay CVs for equine serum samples were 7.34 % and 4.83 % for low (mean: 10.53 µIU/mL) and high concentrations (mean: 109.98 µIU/mL), respectively. The RUD in the first revalidation experiment was 95 % (range from 94 to 96 %), calculated in five dilution steps. The linearity upon dilution was excellent ($r^2 = 0.9994$; $p < 0.0001$), showing a strong relationship between the calculated and measured concentrations of the diluted samples (Fig. 1).

The ELISA provided results within the analytical range for 17 of 20 basal samples and for 11 of 20 stimulated samples (Table 2). The analytical range of the assay was from 2.34 to 175.5 µIU/mL (corresponding range in µg/L: 0.02 to 1.5; conversion factor: 117), as stated by the manufacturer. The mean RUD in samples analyzed by ELISA was 98 ± 4 % (Fig. 2a).

The RIA supplied results for 19 basal samples and for all 20 stimulated samples (Table 2). The analytical range for the RIA was stated as 1.61 to 200.00 µIU/mL. The RUD in the RIA analyses was 160 ± 41 % (Fig. 2b).

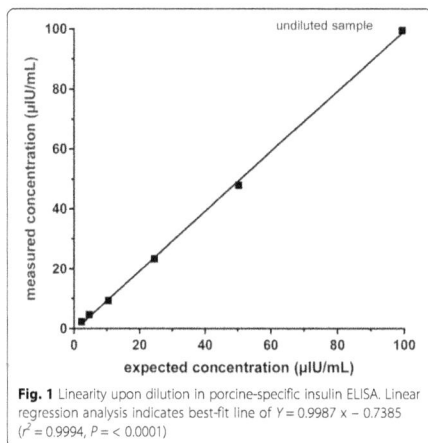

Fig. 1 Linearity upon dilution in porcine-specific insulin ELISA. Linear regression analysis indicates best-fit line of Y = 0.9987 x – 0.7385 ($r^2 = 0.9994$, P = < 0.0001)

Table 2 Information about the number of samples which were measureable within the analytical ranges of the three assays investigated, without previously dilution

Assay	Number of samples	
	Basal, fasted samples	Stimulated OGT samples
ELISA	17/20	11/20
RIA	19/20	20/20
CLIA	20/20	19/20

One of the stimulated samples from the OGT procedure was not measureable within the analytical range (1.0 to 300 µIU/mL) in the CLIA (reported as > 300 µIU/mL) (Table 2). The RUD in the CLIA analyses was 101 ± 11 % (Fig. 2c).

A comparison of the results provided by the three methods of analysis of basal, fasted blood samples for equine insulin indicated statistically significant differences (Fig. 3). Results provided by the CLIA for basal blood samples were significantly ($p < 0.001$) lower compared to results supplied by ELISA or RIA (Fig. 3b, c). Furthermore, differences between ELISA and CLIA in stimulated samples were statistically significant (Fig. 4b), whereas results supplied by ELISA and RIA and RIA and CLIA did not differ significantly (Fig. 4a, c). Despite these differences between insulin concentrations measured by ELISA, RIA and CLIA, Spearman correlations and Deming regression analyses revealed significant correlations and linear relations between all three assays tested (Fig. 5a–c). Bland-Altman Plot analyses showed good agreement with a small bias of −0.44 µIU/mL (95 % limits of agreement: −18.12 to 18.99) comparing the results of ELISA and RIA (Fig. 6a), whereas variations in the results supplied by ELISA compared to CLIA (Fig. 6b; bias: 17.65 µIU/mL; 95 % limits of agreement: −13.92 to 49.22) and CLIA to RIA (Fig. 6c; bias: −8.39 µIU/mL; 95 % limits of agreement: −56.76 to 39.98) occurred. Additionally, the range of variation between results from ELISA and CLIA and between CLIA and RIA increased with elevated insulin concentrations (Fig. 6b, c).

The average recovery rate of equine insulin in 33 samples after one cycle of refreezing and thawing was 97 ± 17 %, but the corresponding range of recovery stretched from 71 to 158 %. In total, insulin concentrations were significantly ($p = 0.0232$) lower in the second measurement (54.99 ± 40.95 µIU/mL) compared to the first (58.5 ± 43.29 µIU/mL). When samples were subdivided into concentration range groups of low (3.51–15.21 µIU/mL), medium (30.42–90.09 µIU/mL) and high (92.43–125.19 µIU/mL) concentrations, the range as well as the mean recovery between the three concentration ranges differed, but there was no statistically significant difference between the first and second measurement when samples were clustered in subgroups depending on concentration. The mean

Warnken *et al. BMC Veterinary Research* (2016) 12:196

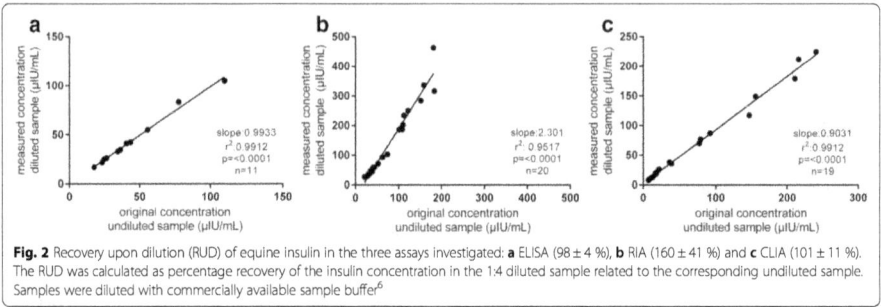

Fig. 2 Recovery upon dilution (RUD) of equine insulin in the three assays investigated: **a** ELISA (98 ± 4 %), **b** RIA (160 ± 41 %) and **c** CLIA (101 ± 11 %). The RUD was calculated as percentage recovery of the insulin concentration in the 1:4 diluted sample related to the corresponding undiluted sample. Samples were diluted with commercially available sample buffer[6]

recovery was 98 ± 16 % (range: 79 to 129 %) in the low, 99 ± 24 % (range: 74 to 158 %) in the medium and 92 ± 12 % (range: 71 to 107 %) in the high concentration group.

Discussion

Most immunoassays used in veterinary medicine for analyzing insulin concentrations in equine serum or plasma samples were originally designed for human diagnostics and research, and specific immunoassays for the quantification of equine insulin are not commercially available. A human-specific insulin radioimmunoassay[8] was used in a variety of equine studies [3, 11, 12] in which several IR and ID diagnostic tests and related reference ranges for plasma and serum insulin had been established. Unfortunately, this assay is no longer available, thus, there is an urgent need to reevaluate the reference ranges established on analyses from samples measured with other approaches for measuring insulin.

Reproducibility, recovery upon dilution and measuring range of assays

The CVs calculated for the ELISA showed that insulin concentration-dependent differences in CVs occurred and

that the CVs calculated by the use of equine serum samples were higher than the CVs stated in the manufacturer's protocol. Very high or low insulin concentrations could not be detected by all assays due to the various analytical ranges of the assays. Therefore, as samples vary greatly in insulin concentration when obtained in fasted conditions or in dynamic diagnostic tests with induced insulin secretion, selection of an assay with an appropriate analytical range is important for the detection of very high or low insulin concentrations. Moreover, our results show that samples with high insulin concentrations, similar to those that can occur in patients with IR or ID, needed to be diluted in some cases to obtain results. Although the ELISA offered the smallest analytical range of the three assays tested, its excellent RUD results enabled the coverage of a broad range of insulin concentrations. Using this ELISA allowed valid measurements of earlier diluted samples of dynamic diagnostic tests. By contrast, using the RIA, all samples could be measured without dilution in the analytical range of the assay. However, RUD experiments did not provide satisfactory results. In a substantial amount of samples, too high insulin concentrations were obtained for the diluted samples compared to the corresponding undiluted samples. The CLIA offered the widest analytical

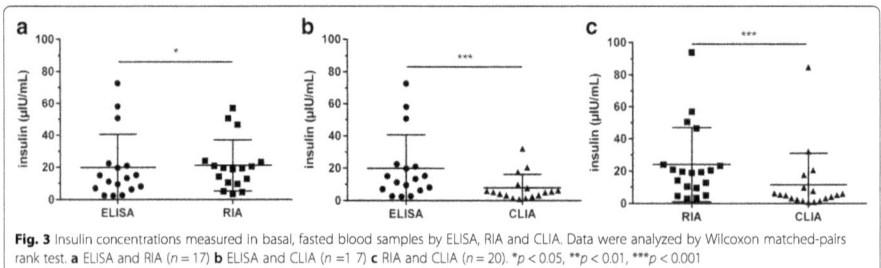

Fig. 3 Insulin concentrations measured in basal, fasted blood samples by ELISA, RIA and CLIA. Data were analyzed by Wilcoxon matched-pairs rank test. **a** ELISA and RIA (n = 17) **b** ELISA and CLIA (n =1 7) **c** RIA and CLIA (n = 20). *p < 0.05, **p < 0.01, ***p < 0.001

MANUSCRIPT I

Warnken *et al. BMC Veterinary Research* (2016) 12:196   Page 6 of 10

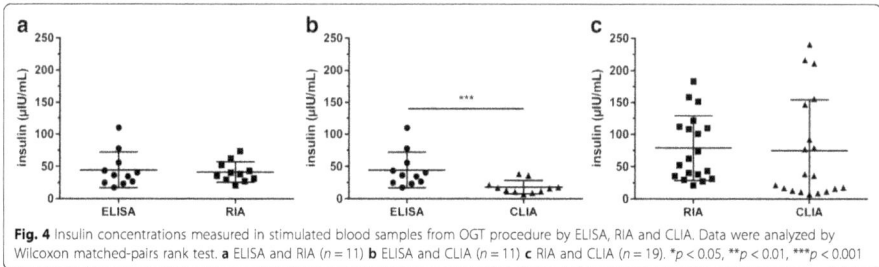

Fig. 4 Insulin concentrations measured in stimulated blood samples from OGT procedure by ELISA, RIA and CLIA. Data were analyzed by Wilcoxon matched-pairs rank test. **a** ELISA and RIA (*n* = 11) **b** ELISA and CLIA (*n* = 11) **c** RIA and CLIA (*n* = 19). *p < 0.05, **p < 0.01, ***p < 0.001

range when compared to the other two assays, but also could not measure all high insulin concentration samples. This assay, similar to the ELISA, exhibited good RUD results, leading to the conclusion that appropriate dilution of samples in this assay do not falsify results.

Dilution buffers

We used commercially available sample buffer[6] to dilute the samples in this study. This buffer was designed for use in the ELISA investigated. Öberg and colleagues [8] evaluated the RUD and linearity of dilution in this ELISA with physiologic saline as a dilution medium in four dilution steps and found similar results regarding linearity, but poorer RUD of 92 to 122 %. Dilution of serum samples with zero calibrator provided in the ELISA yielded higher recovery rates of 102.4 ± 20.5 % in another study [13]. Therefore, dilution of samples with the manufacturer's commercially available sample buffer[6] seems to improve results obtained from diluted samples in this assay. Tinworth and colleagues [6] recommended that samples with high insulin concentrations which required dilution should be diluted with charcoal stripped equine plasma instead of the manufacturer's diluent in order to improve results obtained by analysis with a human-specific insulin RIA[8] mentioned previously. One

limitation in our study is that all our samples have been diluted with commercially available sample buffer[6] designed for use in the equine-optimized, porcine-specific ELISA and were then used in the different assays. Therefore, results of this RUD analysis may also be impaired by interactions of the dilution medium and assay components. The RUD results may be improved by using an appropriate method-dependent dilution medium.

Insulin molecule stability

The stability of insulin in blood samples is a commonly discussed issue in both human and veterinary medicine. Optimal pre-analytical handling of samples is essential for valid analytical results, but is often not feasible in the daily routine of an ambulatory practice. The recovery range observed indicates quite variable results. Some of the refrozen and thawed samples measured had a lower insulin concentration in the second analysis, whereas others had higher insulin concentrations. Parts of the variations and effects between the first and second measurement may be due to inter-assay variations, but, as already presented, inter-assay CVs for low equine insulin concentration samples and high insulin concentration samples in the ELISA were within the generally accepted variation range for immunoassays [14]. A study

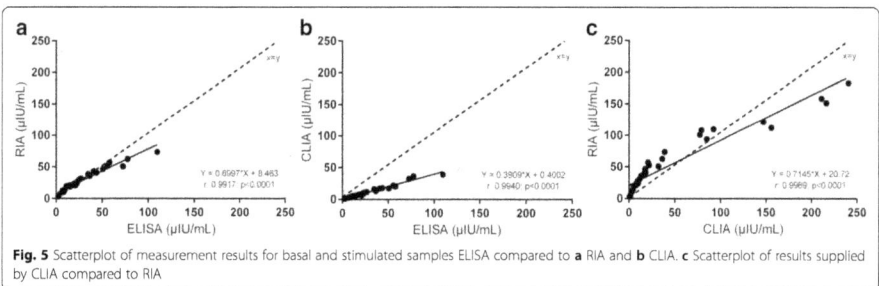

Fig. 5 Scatterplot of measurement results for basal and stimulated samples ELISA compared to **a** RIA and **b** CLIA. **c** Scatterplot of results supplied by CLIA compared to RIA

MANUSCRIPT I

Warnken *et al. BMC Veterinary Research* (2016) 12:196　　　　　　　　　　　Page 7 of 10

a
difference (µIU/mL)
100
50
0
-50
-100
50 ··· 100 ··· 150 ··· 200
average (µIU/mL)

b
difference (µIU/mL)
100
50
0
-50
-100
50 ··· 100 ··· 150 ··· 200
average (µIU/mL)

c
difference (µIU/mL)
100
50
0
-50
-100
50 100 150 200 250
average (µIU/mL)

Fig. 6 Bland-Altman plot of average compared to difference **a** ELISA minus RIA (*n* = 28), **b** ELISA minus CLIA (*n* = 28) and **c** CLIA minus RIA (*n* = 39). Dashed line = bias, pointed line = 95 % limits of agreements

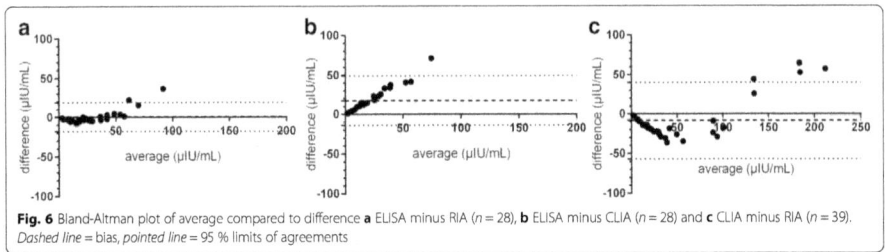

by Livesey and colleagues [15] indicated that repeated thawing and freezing affected the insulin concentration in human plasma samples collected during intravenous glucose tolerance testing procedures. Insulin concentrations had already declined after the first freezing and thawing cycle and exhibited a continuous decline during following freezing and thawing cycles. A more recent study by Mechanic and colleagues [16] examined the effect of short-term refrigerated storage at ≤ −70 °C on insulin in human blood samples and found no significant effect in a time period of 72 h and also no significant effect of delays in freezing following centrifugation 2 h post-collection, whereas they observed declined insulin concentrations following delays in centrifugation. Furthermore, repeated freezing and thawing of serum did not affect the concentrations of insulin in serum samples from beagle dogs [17]. Borer-Weier and colleagues [13] evaluated the stability of equine insulin after freezing and thawing in their study and showed similar results to our study, with large ranges of differences in the samples analyzed with human-specific RIA[8] and a high-range porcine insulin ELISA. One limitation in our study design, as well as in other previous studies, was that serum insulin concentrations were not measured directly after the sampling procedure, prior to first freezing, so the effect of the first, initial freeze remains unknown. Taking into account the variable effects of freezing and thawing on the insulin concentrations in the samples we analyzed, we recommend that samples are not frozen and thawed any more than necessary in order not to receive false results.

Conversion factors for insulin measures
Various conversion factors have been established in the past due to the differences in insulin binding efficacy. Data had to be converted from µg/L into the commonly used SI unit µIU/mL to compare the results from ELISA with results derived from RIA and CLIA. In previous studies in which insulin analysis had been performed with the equine-optimized porcine-specific ELISA, data was either presented in µg/L [9, 10, 18] or converted into mU/L [19]. In the latter case, conversion was performed

without an exact statement regarding the conversion factor, which was suggested to be 10 in an earlier publication by the same author [9]. In addition, the factor 28.69 (1 µg/L = 28.69 for µIU/mL) [20] for the conversion of human insulin was discussed. However, for the ELISA used in our study, the cross-reactivity with the human insulin molecule is only 22 %, as declared by the manufacturer. Therefore, the use of both factors for conversion of the data generated by the equine-optimized, porcine-specific ELISA might be questionable. Thus, another equine-specific conversion factor (1 µg/L = 117 mU/L) was given by the manufacturer for this assay [21] and was used for the calculation of data in our study.

Comparison of methods and assay insulin antibodies
Equine insulin has a lower molecular weight (5.748 kDa) compared to human (5.808 kDa) and porcine insulin (5.778 kDa) and consists of 51 amino acids. The equine insulin differs from the human and porcine insulin molecule in the amino acid sequence [22, 23]. Even slight differences in the amino acid sequences between species and, thus, secondary structure can result in impaired antibody binding and can, therefore, cause variations in efficacy when measuring insulin by different immunoassay-based methods. Comparing the results of converted data, all three methods provided different insulin concentrations within the same samples. The CLIA results observed in this study were markedly lower than the results supplied by the ELISA and the RIA. Data analyses with Bland-Altman plots and Deming regression analyses indicated that there was no constant systemic error, meaning that one method measures consistently higher or lower than the other ones. The ELISA supplied higher insulin concentrations than the CLIA and the difference between both methods even increased with rising concentrations, indicating the presence of proportional error. The CLIA also provided lower results than the RIA for samples with concentrations under 100 µIU/mL, but when the concentration exceeded 100 µIU/mL, the CLIA supplied higher results for five samples compared to the RIA. These differences between

38

Warnken et al. BMC Veterinary Research (2016) 12:196

insulin concentration results provided by the three assays may be caused by underlying antibodies used in the different assays. The ELISA and the RIA were based on antibodies directed against porcine insulin, which differs in amino acid 9 of the A chain (glycine in equine insulin and serine in porcine insulin), whereas human and equine insulin differ in amino acid 9 on the A chain and amino acid 30 of the B chain (alanine in equine insulin and threonine in human insulin) [22]. Differences at amino acid 9 on the A chain are not considered to be important for biological activity, but changes in amino acid 30 on the B chain were discussed to affect the 3D structure [23, 24]. Therefore, the markedly lower results provided by the CLIA may be caused by a loss of homology in this position and variation in 3D structure, which may impair sufficient antigen-antibody binding by steric interference. Furthermore, alterations in the antigenic epitope for the anti-human insulin antibody used in the CLIA may cause insufficient antigen-antibody binding. Variations in insulin concentrations, such as occurred in our study, have already been described by several authors for other assays and methods used frequently. Tinworth and colleagues [6] compared the equine-optimized, porcine-specific insulin ELISA and a modified version of the human-specific RIA[8] in their investigations. Both assays gave different insulin concentration results for the same samples as well, and underestimated the insulin concentration compared to liquid chromatography and high-resolution/high-accuracy mass spectrometry (LC-MS) [6]. The LC-MS provides absolute amounts of insulin and could be assessed as a gold standard to measure insulin concentrations in blood samples. Due to a lack of LC-MS in our study, potential over- or underestimation of the assays examined could not be evaluated. Banse and colleagues [7] compared the human-specific RIA[8] with another commercially available CLIA[9] which is often used for the measurement of equine insulin in both clinical practice and research. Both the human-specific RIA[8] and the CLIA[9] resulted in poor recovery rates within each assay and showed poor accordance. They, furthermore, examined the recovery of equine insulin standard within both assays. The recovery rate was poor in both assays, but the CLIA[9] investigated showed recovery rates of only up to 10 %. However, no equine insulin standard was available in our experiments; therefore, we could not examine the equine insulin standard recovery in the three immunoassays investigated in this study.

Clinical relevance of valid insulin measures

The clinical relevance of result variation becomes obvious when focusing on basal samples. According to the current state in equine veterinary practice, analysis of basal samples from fasted patients as a screening method for IR and ID accounts for a large proportion of insulin measurements in

veterinary diagnostics. In veterinary practice, basal insulin concentrations of 20 μIU/mL were stated as cut-off values to distinguish between healthy and insulin-resistant or insulin-dysregulated horses in the consensus statements of the American College of Veterinary Internal Medicine [12]. On closer inspection, this cut-off value was suggested as being valid for sample analyses resting upon the Coat-A-Count insulin radioimmunoassay[8] (Siemens Medical Solutions Diagnostics, Los Angeles, CA), Immulite insulin solid-phase chemiluminescent assay[9] (Siemens Medical Solutions Diagnostics) and DSL-1600 insulin radioimmunoassay (Diagnostic Systems Laboratory Inc, Webster, TX) by the authors of the consensus statement. However, this cut-off value is often used without consideration of the underlying analysis method. Thus, assay-dependent differences in the insulin concentration levels measured can cause false classification of patients. Calculations of indices, which are based on basal insulin and glucose concentrations for estimation of IR, were used more commonly [25] and, therefore, could result in false diagnosis of IR. Exact differentiation between 15 and 30 μIU/mL may be very important for the interpretation of basal samples. In six of the seventeen animals investigated, analysis of basal, fasted blood samples by the three assays investigated led to different classification as insulin-sensitive or insulin-dysregulated depending on the data used. One of our samples illustrates this problem. The CLIA supplied an insulin concentration of 7.8 μIU/mL, whereupon this horse is classified as insulin-sensitive when considering the cut-off value of 20 μIU/mL recommended by the American College of Veterinary Internal Medicine. By contrast, ELISA and RIA supplied insulin concentrations of 50.73 μIU/mL and 46.53 μIU/mL, respectively, after which this horse is classified as insulin-resistant or insulin-dysregulated on the basis of basal, fasted blood analysis. Both commercial laboratories we commissioned with the analyses of our samples provided laboratory-specific reference values for insulin in fasted serum blood samples of horses. The reference range stated for the RIA was < 20 μIU/mL in fasted samples and was < 23.4 μIU/mL for the CLIA. These findings indicate that even consideration of laboratory and assay-specific reference ranges leads to different classification of this horse, depending on the assay used to determine the basal, fasted blood insulin concentration. As a consequence, independent of laboratory and assay-specific reference ranges or cut-off values, a general harmonization of equine insulin analyses is urgently required to allow accurate and safe diagnosis of hyperinsulinemia as one of the leading symptoms in horses suffering from EMS.

Conclusion

In conclusion, analyses of equine serum samples for insulin with three different immunoassay methods revealed

MANUSCRIPT I

Warnken et al. BMC Veterinary Research (2016) 12:196
Page 9 of 10

three different results for the same sample. Adjustment of insulin measurements and methods is essential to allow the consistence of information of several studies and research approaches, enabling evidence-based criteria to compare insulin concentrations consistently between assays, studies and laboratories. Since harmonization is an interminable process, further assay comparison research studies would be helpful to allow the comparison of results and cut-off values determined with the use of one method to another. This study illustrates the importance of considering the insulin analysis method when results of different laboratories or studies are compared or interpreted for the diagnosis of insulin-related endocrine and metabolic pathologies.

Endnotes

[1]Equine Insulin ELISA, Mercodia AB, Uppsala, Sweden.
[2]Porcine Insulin RIA, Millipore, St. Charles, MO, USA.
[3]ADVIA Centaur Insulin Assay, Siemens Healthcare Diagnostics Gmbh, Eschborn, Germany.
[4]Vacuette® Greiner Bio One, Frickenhausen, Germany.
[5]Animal Insulin Control, 362 Mercodia AB, Uppsala, Sweden.
[6]Diabetes Sample Buffer, Mercodia AB, Uppsala, Sweden.
[7]Graphpad Prism, Version 6.02 for Windows, Graph-Pad Inc. La Jolla, CA, USA.
[8]Coat-a-Count Insulin RIA, Siemens Medical Solutions Diagnostics, Los Angeles, CA, USA.
[9]Immulite Insulin Assay, Siemens Healthcare, Malvern, PA, USA.

Abbreviations
CV: Coefficient of variation; EMS: Equine metabolic syndrome; Fig: Figure; ID: Insulin dysregulation; IR: Insulin resistance; ELISA: Enzyme-linked immunosorbent assay; RIA: Radioimmunoassay; CLIA: Chemiluminescent immunoassay; RUD: Recovery upon dilution; LC-MS: Liquid chromatography and high-resolution/high-accuracy mass spectrometry; SD: Standard deviation; Tab: Table

Acknowledgements
The authors are grateful for financial support from Boehringer Ingelheim Vetmedica Gmbh. Furthermore the authors thank Mrs. Kathrin Hansen for technical support in the laboratory and language editor Philip Saunders for the validation of the English language used in this article.

Funding
This research was financially supported by Boehringer-Ingelheim-Vetmedica Gmbh.

Availability of data and materials
Data and materials are available upon request.

Authors' contributions
TW, KH and KF designed the study. TW collected and analyzed data, wrote the manuscript and made figures. KH and KF helped to edit the manuscript. All authors read and approved the final manuscript.

Competing interests
The authors declare that they have no competing interests.

Consent for publication
Not applicable.

Ethics approval and consent to participate
Samples from university-owned control horses had been obtained during a study which has been approved by the ethics committee within the University of Veterinary Medicine, Hannover, and the State Office for Consumer Protection and Food Safety in accordance with the German Animal Welfare Law (LAVES– Reference number: 33.14 42502-04-13/1259). Samples from insulin dysregulated horses and ponies were collected during routine diagnostic procedures in the Clinic for Horses and owners provided informed consent that samples can be included in the study.

Author details
[1]Department of Physiology, University of Veterinary Medicine Hannover, Foundation, Bischofsholer Damm 15, 30173 Hannover, Germany. [2]Institute of Animal Science, Faculty of Agricultural Sciences, University of Hohenheim, Fruwirthstraße 35, 70593 Stuttgart, Germany. [3]Clinic for Horses, University of Veterinary Medicine Hannover, Foundation, Bünteweg 9, 30559 Hannover, Germany.

Received: 26 February 2016 Accepted: 1 September 2016
Published online: 09 September 2016

References
1. Schuver A, Frank N, Chameroy KA, Elliott SB. Assessment of insulin and glucose dynamics by using an oral sugar test in horses. J Equine Vet Sci. 2014;34:465–70.
2. Ralston SL. Insulin and glucose regulation. Vet Clin North Am Equine Pract. 2002;18:295–304.
3. Eiler H, Frank N, Andrews FM, Oliver JW, Fecteau KA. Physiologic assessment of blood glucose homeostasis via combined intravenous glucose and insulin testing in horses. Am J Vet Res. 2005;66:1598–604.
4. Rijnen KE, van der Kolk JH. Determination of reference range values indicative of glucose metabolism and insulin resistance by use of glucose clamp techniques in horses and ponies. Am J Vet Res. 2003;64:1260–4.
5. Frank N, Tadros EM. Insulin dysregulation. Equine Vet J. 2014;46:103–12.
6. Tinworth KD, Wynn PC, Boston RC, Harris PA, Sillence MN, Thevis M, Thomas A, Noble GK. Evaluation of commercially available assays for the measurement of equine insulin. Domest Anim Endocrinol. 2011;41:81–90.
7. Banse HE, McCann J, Yang F, Wagg C, McFarlane D. Comparison of two methods for measurement of equine insulin. J Vet Diagn Invest. 2014;26:527–30.
8. Öberg J, Bröjer J, Wattle O, Lilliehöök I. Evaluation of an equine-optimized enzyme-linked immunosorbent assay for serum insulin measurement and stability study of equine serum insulin. Comp Clin Path. 2011;21:1291–300.
9. Brojer JT, Nostell KE, Essen-Gustavsson B, Hedenstrom UO. Effect of repeated oral administration of glucose and leucine immediately after exercise on plasma insulin concentration and glycogen synthesis in horses. Am J Vet Res. 2012;73:867–74.
10. Brunner J, Wichert B, Burger D, von Peinen K, Liesegang A. A survey on the feeding of eventing horses during competition. J Anim Physiol Anim Nutr (Berl). 2012;96:878–84.
11. Frank N, Elliott SB, Brandt LE, Keisler DH. Physical characteristics, blood hormone concentrations, and plasma lipid concentrations in obese horses with insulin resistance. J Am Vet Med Assoc. 2006;228:1383–90.
12. Frank N, Geor RJ, Bailey SR, Durham AE, Johnson PJ, American College of Veterinary Internal M. Equine metabolic syndrome. J Vet Intern Med. 2010;24:467–75.
13. Borer-Weir KE, Bailey SR, Menzies-Gow NJ, Harris PA, Elliott J. Evaluation of a commercially available radioimmunoassay and species-specific ELISAs for measurement of high concentrations of insulin in equine serum. Amn J Vet Res. 2012;73:1596–602.
14. European Medicines Agency: Guideline on bioanalytical method validation. 2011. http://www.ema.europa.eu/docs/en_GB/document_library/Scientific_guideline/2011/08/WC500109686.pdf. Accessed 21 Jan 2016.
15. Livesey JH, Hodgkinson SC, Roud HR, Donald RA. Effect of time, temperature and freezing on the stability of immunoreactive LH, FSH, TSH, growth hormone, prolactin and insulin in plasma. Clin Biochem. 1980;13:151–5.

MANUSCRIPT I

Warnken *et al. BMC Veterinary Research* (2016) 12:196

Page 10 of 10

16. Mechanic L, Mendez A, Merrill L, Rogers J, Layton M, Todd D, Varanasi A, O'Brien B, Meyer Iii WA, Zhang M, et al. Planned variation in preanalytical conditions to evaluate biospecimen stability in the National Children's Study (NCS). Clin Chem Lab Med. 2013;51:2287–94.
17. Reimers TJ, McCann JP, Cowan RG, Concannon PW. Effects of storage, hemolysis, and freezing and thawing on concentrations of thyroxine, cortisol, and insulin in blood samples. Proc Soc Exp Biol Med. 1982;170:509–16.
18. Nostell KE, Essen-Gustavsson B, Brojer JT. Repeated post-exercise administration with a mixture of leucine and glucose alters the plasma amino acid profile in Standardbred trotters. Acta Vet Scand. 2012;54:7.
19. Brojer J, Lindase S, Hedenskog J, Alvarsson K, Nostell K. Repeatability of the combined glucose-insulin tolerance test and the effect of a stressor before testing in horses of 2 breeds. J Vet Intern Med. 2013;27:1543–50.
20. Volund A. Conversion of insulin units to SI units. Am J Clin Nutr. 1993;58:714–5.
21. Mercodia AB. Technical Note No: 34–0128. How to compare insulin values between mU/L and μg/L when using Mercodia Insulin ELISAs (Version 1.0). https://www.mercodia.com. Acessed 17 Feb 2015.
22. Ho EN, Wan TS, Wong AS, Lam KK, Stewart BD. Doping control analysis of insulin and its analogues in equine plasma by liquid chromatography-tandem mass spectrometry. J Chromatogr A. 2008;1201:183–90.
23. Kuuranne T, Thomas A, Leinonen A, Delahaut P, Bosseloir A, Schanzer W, Thevis M. Insulins in equine urine: qualitative analysis by immunoaffinity purification and liquid chromatography/tandem mass spectrometry for doping control purposes in horse-racing. Rapid Commun Mass Spectrom. 2008;22:355–62.
24. Conlon JM. Evolution of the insulin molecule: insights into structure-activity and phylogenetic relationships. Peptides. 2001;22:1183–93.
25. Treiber KH, Kronfeld DS, Hess TM, Boston RC, Harris PA. Use of proxies and reference quintiles obtained from minimal model analysis for determination of insulin sensitivity and pancreatic beta-cell responsiveness in horses. Am J Vet Res. 2005;66:2114–21.

6 PART II – MANUSCRIPT II

Retrospective analysis of insulin responses to standard dosed oral glucose tests (Ogts) via naso-gastric tubing towards definition of an objective cut-off value

Tobias Warnken[1*], Julien Delarocque[1], Svenja Schumacher[1], Korinna Huber[2], Karsten Feige[1]

[1] Clinic for Horses, University of Veterinary Medicine Hannover, Foundation, Bünteweg 9, 30559 Hannover, Germany

[2] Institute of Animal Science, Faculty of Agricultural Sciences, University of Hohenheim, Fruwirthstraße 35, 70599 Stuttgart, Germany

*Corresponding author: Tobias Warnken

Acta Veterinaria Scandinavica 2018; 60(1):4

Accepted: 14th January 2018, available online: 19th January 2018.

DOI: 10.1186/s13028-018-0358-8

https://actavetscand.biomedcentral.com/articles/10.1186/s13028-018-0358-8

Contribution to the manuscript

TW and KF designed the study. TW and SS collected data. TW and JD analyzed data, wrote the manuscript and made figures. KH and KF helped to edit the manuscript. All authors read and approved the final manuscript.

Abstract

Background: Insulin dysregulation (ID) with basal or postprandial hyperinsulinemia is one of the key findings in horses and ponies suffering from the equine metabolic syndrome (EMS). Assessment of ID can easily be performed in clinical settings by the use of oral glucose challenge tests. Oral glucose test (OGT) performed with 1 g/kg bodyweight (BW) glucose administered via naso-gastric tube allows the exact administration of a defined glucose dosage in a short time. However, reliable cut-off values have not been available so far. Therefore, the aim of the study was to describe variations in insulin response to OGT via naso-gastric tubing and to provide a clinical useful cut-off value for ID when using the insulin quantification performed with an equine-optimized insulin enzyme-linked immunosorbent assay.

Results: Data visualization revealed no clear separation in the serum insulin concentration of insulin sensitive and insulin dysregulated horses during OGT. Therefore, a model based clustering method was used to circumvent the use of an arbitrary limit for categorization. This method considered all data-points for the classification, taking into account the individual insulin trajectory during the OGT. With this method two clusters were differentiated, one with low and one with high insulin responses during OGT. The cluster of individuals with low insulin response was consistently detected, independently of the initialization parameters of the algorithm. In this cluster the 97.5% quantile of insulin is 110 µIU/mL at 120 min. We suggest using this insulin concentration of 110 µIU/mL as a cut-off value for samples obtained at 120 min in OGT.

Conclusion: OGT performed with 1 g/kg BW glucose and administration via naso-gastric tubing can easily be performed under clinical settings. Application of the cut-off value of 110 µIU/mL at 120 min allows assessment of ID in horses.

Keywords: ELISA, Equine metabolic syndrome, Horse, Insulin, Insulin dysregulation, Naso-gastric tubing, Oral glucose test

Warnken *et al. Acta Vet Scand* (2018) 60:4
https://doi.org/10.1186/s13028-018-0358-8

Acta Veterinaria Scandinavica

Retrospective analysis of insulin responses to standard dosed oral glucose tests (OGTs) via naso-gastric tubing towards definition of an objective cut-off value

Tobias Warnken[1*], Julien Delarocque[1], Svenja Schumacher[1], Korinna Huber[2] and Karsten Feige[1]

Abstract

Background: Insulin dysregulation (ID) with basal or postprandial hyperinsulinemia is one of the key findings in horses and ponies suffering from the equine metabolic syndrome (EMS). Assessment of ID can easily be performed in clinical settings by the use of oral glucose challenge tests. Oral glucose test (OGT) performed with 1 g/kg bodyweight (BW) glucose administered via naso-gastric tube allows the exact administration of a defined glucose dosage in a short time. However, reliable cut-off values have not been available so far. Therefore, the aim of the study was to describe variations in insulin response to OGT via naso-gastric tubing and to provide a clinical useful cut-off value for ID when using the insulin quantification performed with an equine-optimized insulin enzyme-linked immunosorbent assay.

Results: Data visualization revealed no clear separation in the serum insulin concentration of insulin sensitive and insulin dysregulated horses during OGT. Therefore, a model based clustering method was used to circumvent the use of an arbitrary limit for categorization. This method considered all data-points for the classification, taking into account the individual insulin trajectory during the OGT. With this method two clusters were differentiated, one with low and one with high insulin responses during OGT. The cluster of individuals with low insulin response was consistently detected, independently of the initialization parameters of the algorithm. In this cluster the 97.5% quantile of insulin is 110 µLU/mL at 120 min. We suggest using this insulin concentration of 110 µLU/mL as a cut-off value for samples obtained at 120 min in OGT.

Conclusion: OGT performed with 1 g/kg BW glucose and administration via naso-gastric tubing can easily be performed under clinical settings. Application of the cut-off value of 110 µLU/mL at 120 min allows assessment of ID in horses.

Keywords: ELISA, Equine metabolic syndrome, Horse, Insulin, Insulin dysregulation, Naso-gastric tubing, Oral glucose test

Findings

The equine metabolic syndrome (EMS) is a common endocrinopathy in equines. Horses are affected by general or regional obesity, predisposition to laminitis and insulin dysregulation (ID). Insulin dysregulation refers to basal and/or postprandial hyperinsulinemia, sometimes

also associated with tissue insulin resistance [1, 2]. Moreover, ID can occur in EMS as well as in pituitary *pars intermedia* dysfunction (PPID) patients [3, 4]. Unfortunately, ID horses may not be identified correctly by phenotype in all cases. Furthermore, baseline measurements of fasting glucose and insulin concentrations may not suffice in all patients [1, 5]. Therefore, dynamic tests are proposed for the assessment of ID [1, 2, 6, 7].

Oral glucose challenge tests allow assessment of postprandial hyperinsulinemia in ID horses under

---
*Correspondence: tobias.warnken@tiho-hannover.de
[1] Clinic for Horses, University of Veterinary Medicine Hannover, Foundation, Bünteweg 9, 30559 Hannover, Germany
Full list of author information is available at the end of the article

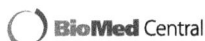

MANUSCRIPT II

Warnken *et al. Acta Vet Scand (2018) 60:4*   Page 2 of 5

standardized conditions. Recently published research highlights the importance of hyperinsulinemia, reporting that laminitis can be induced experimentally using a diet high in nonstructural carbohydrates. Furthermore, the authors were able to predict laminitis risk based on insulin and glucose levels after an oral challenge test [8]. Several oral test protocols for assessment of ID are currently available. In these procedures application routes as well as the used dosages of glucose or other sugars vary. The in-feed oral glucose tests (OGT) can be performed by feeding 0.5 g–1.0 g/kg bodyweight (BW) glucose or dextrose powder mixed in low-glycemic meals and by determination of insulin and glucose concentrations after 120 min [9]. A positive test and ID was defined as an insulin concentration > 80 μLU/mL [1] or > 87 μLU/mL [10], depending on which literature is consulted. The oral sugar test (OST) as a simplified testing procedure uses 0.15 mL/kg BW corn syrup [11] administered orally via syringe, followed by measurement of insulin and glucose after 75 min. Insulin concentrations > 60 μLU/mL were used as cut-off [10, 12]. Recently, a dosage of 0.25 mL/kg BW for OST was suggested to improve diagnostic value. Blood sample analysis was recommended at either 60, 75, 90 or 120 min and insulin concentrations of $\geq$ 22.8, 18.7, 30.2 and 26.3 μLU/mL, respectively were proposed for being indicative for ID [13]. Since corn syrup is not available in most European countries, a modified OST using commercially available Scandinavian glucose syrup was developed and provided promising results [14]. Nevertheless, reference ranges have not been established to date. Moreover, clinicians and researchers reported acceptance problems in their patients when performing in-feed OGTs, which led to prolonged consumption times or refused feed intake and therefore precluded reliable and exact test results for interpretation [15].

An alternative is to perform the OGT via naso-gastric tubing [16]. The substantial benefit of this protocol is the exact administration of a defined glucose dosage in a short time. Though it remains the most precise oral test approach, this procedure requires naso-gastric tubing. For OGT performed with 1 g/kg BW glucose dissolved in 2 L water and administration via naso-gastric tubing, there are no reliable cut-off values or reference ranges available. Therefore, the aim of the study was to describe variations in insulin response to OGT via naso-gastric tubing and to provide a clinical useful cut-off value for ID when using insulin quantification performed with an equine-optimized insulin enzyme-linked immunosorbent assay (ELISA).[1]

OGT results of 56 horses and ponies were obtained under similar conditions during several research projects from winter 2013 to spring 2017. Twenty-three warmblood horses, 19 Icelandic horses, 5 Shetland ponies and 9 ponies of various breeds were included in the study regardless of their insulin sensitivity status. There were 26 mares, 25 geldings and 5 stallions, aged 15 ± 6 years and weighed 473 ± 136 kg. The included horses had a mean body condition score (BCS) of 5.9 ± 1.4. Out of 56 individuals 16 were previously diagnosed with laminitis. OGTs were performed under standardized conditions after 12–14 h fasting prior to testing.

To perform OGT, 1 g/kg BW glucose powder[2] was dissolved in 2 L of water and administered via naso-gastric tubing [16]. Blood samples were collected via intravenous catheter[3,4] prior to administration of the glucose solution, and afterwards in 15 min intervals for at least 180 min. Blood samples for serum preparation were placed into plain tubes, incubated at room temperature, centrifuged after 60 min at $1000 \times g$ for 6 min, and stored at − 80 °C until further analysis. Serum insulin concentrations were analyzed in duplicate using an equine-optimized insulin ELISA (see footnote 1) previously validated for use in horses [17, 18]. Samples with insulin concentrations exceeding the analytical range of the ELISA (> 1.5 μg/L) were diluted with commercially available sample buffer.[5] For the conversion of insulin concentrations expressed in μg/L as supplied by the ELISA, to the commonly used SI unit of μLU/mL, the previously published conversion factor of 115 was used [19].

Statistical analysis was performed in R 3.4.0.[6] Dynamics in insulin responses to OGT showed large variation in the study population ruling out simple visual differentiation between two groups of insulin sensitive and insulin dysregulated animals (Fig. 1). Moreover, there is no clear separation in the serum insulin concentration of insulin sensitive and insulin dysregulated horses at the currently used time-point for evaluation of 120 min in the OGT. Therefore, data analysis was performed using a model based clustering method provided by the mclust R-package [20] in combination with a scaled singular value decomposition (SVD) projection for improved initialization [21]. This algorithm tries to detect an intrinsic structure to the data in an unsupervised manner by grouping individuals based on their similarities in insulin measurements at all sampling time points. The benefits are that no arbitrary limit is used for categorization and that all

---

[2] Glukose, WDT, Garbsen, Germany.

[3] EquiCath^{TM} Fastflow, 12 G, Braun Vet Care GmbH, Tuttlingen, Germany.

[4] Intraflon 2, 12 G, Vygon, Ecouen, France.

[5] Diabetes Sample Buffer, Mercodia AB, Uppsala, Sweden.

[6] R version 3.4.0, The R Foundation for Statistical Computing.

---

[1] Equine Insulin ELISA, Mercodia AB, Uppsala, Sweden.

MANUSCRIPT II

Warnken et al. Acta Vet Scand (2018) 60:4

Page 3 of 5

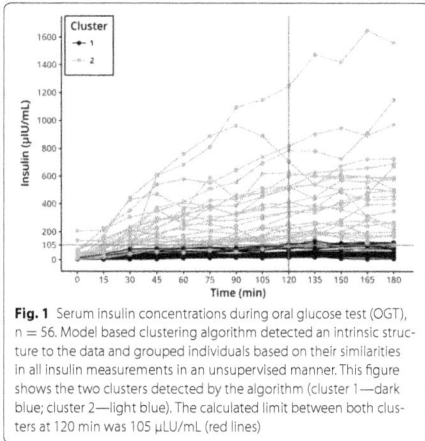

Fig. 1 Serum insulin concentrations during oral glucose test (OGT), n = 56. Model based clustering algorithm detected an intrinsic structure to the data and grouped individuals based on their similarities in all insulin measurements in an unsupervised manner. This figure shows the two clusters detected by the algorithm (cluster 1—dark blue; cluster 2—light blue). The calculated limit between both clusters at 120 min was 105 µLU/mL (red lines)

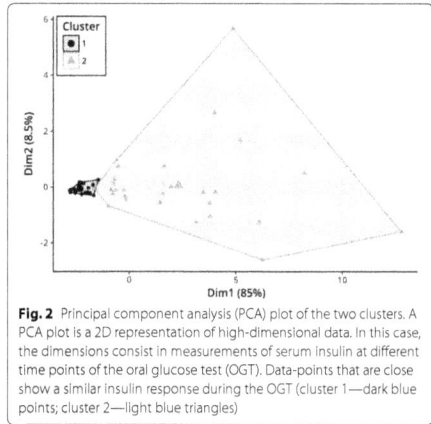

Fig. 2 Principal component analysis (PCA) plot of the two clusters. A PCA plot is a 2D representation of high-dimensional data. In this case, the dimensions consist in measurements of serum insulin at different time points of the oral glucose test (OGT). Data-points that are close show a similar insulin response during the OGT (cluster 1—dark blue points; cluster 2—light blue triangles)

data-points are used in the classification, taking into account the individual insulin response during the OGT. The clustering results were compared with other clustering methods like partitioning (kmeans, pam) and hierarchical clustering with varying initialization parameters. A cluster with constant lower insulin concentrations during the OGT (cluster 1) was consistently found across the different clustering strategies, while the optimal number of clusters varied. The model based clustering approach was preferred because it required no a priori estimation of the number of clusters. Two clusters retained by the mclust algorithm with improved initialization relate to another (Figs. 1, 2). The separation line between the two clusters at 120 min was at 105 µLU/L insulin. As the serum insulin in each group for each time-point did not belong to a normal distribution, the (pseudo) median was of more informative value than the mean. Figure 3 shows the pseudomedian with 95% confidence interval for both clusters as estimated from the Hodges-Lehmann estimator. While the difference between groups was striking, the actual range of insulin responses that occurred in different subjects supports the idea that insulin status is not a dichotomous state of either insulin sensitive or insulin dysregulated but rather that ID exists in different intensities (Fig. 1). For calculation of a reliable cut-off value, 97.5% quantile of the cluster 1 constituted a cut-off of 110 µLU/mL insulin at 120 min (Fig. 4). With respect to previously reported significant differences between laboratory methods used for quantification of equine insulin [18, 22, 23], our reported cut-off value is only applicable for the combination of the OGT procedure described

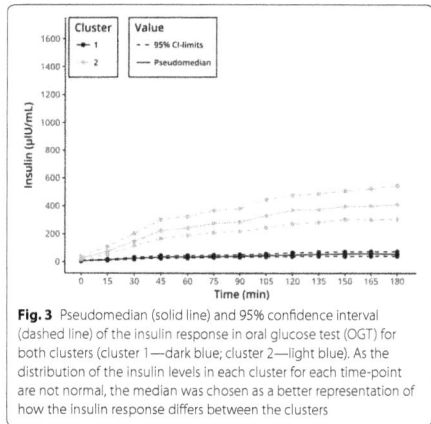

Fig. 3 Pseudomedian (solid line) and 95% confidence interval (dashed line) of the insulin response in oral glucose test (OGT) for both clusters (cluster 1—dark blue; cluster 2—light blue). As the distribution of the insulin levels in each cluster for each time-point are not normal, the median was chosen as a better representation of how the insulin response differs between the clusters

above and the measurement of insulin by the use of the equine-optimized ELISA (see footnote 1) or a method which shows good agreement. However, even intra- and inter-assay CV values of 2.0–10.6% and 4.83–10.7% reported for the immunoassay used in this study can impair final results [17, 18, 24]. Sixteen horses of the study population had radiographically confirmed laminitis. Fifteen out of sixteen laminitic horses and ponies were positively identified as ID by this OGT when the cut-off value of 110 µLU/mL was applied. Moreover, the median (IQR) insulin concentration of previously

MANUSCRIPT II

Warnken *et al. Acta Vet Scand (2018) 60:4*   Page 4 of 5

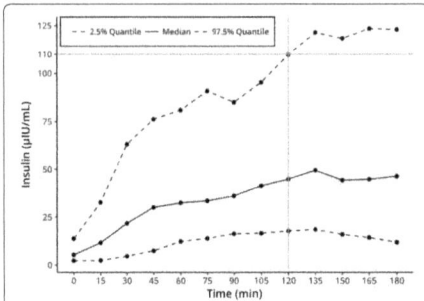

Fig. 4 Median serum insulin concentration (solid line) of the cluster 1 classified as insulin sensitive during oral glucose test (OGT) with calculated 2.5 and 97.5% quantile (dashed lines). Calculated cut-off at 120 min is 110 µLU/mL (grey lines)

laminitic individuals was 513.3 (187.6–618.9) µLU/mL at 120 min during OGT. This is the first study providing a cut-off for OGT performed with 1 g/kg BW glucose administered via naso-gastric tube. Nevertheless, insulin concentrations around 110 µLU/mL should be interpreted carefully in clinical situations in which significant management and feeding modifications or even drug therapies would be initiated when patients are classified as insulin dysregulated. In these cases with debatable insulin concentrations following OGT, re-testing horses and ponies after a certain period of time would be advisable. The authors suggest not using the reported value as a strict cut-off, but rather as an orientation value for clinical interpretation and diagnosing ID because of the fluent transition between horses and ponies with undisturbed insulin regulation and ID.

Taking into account the reported coefficient of variation (CV) values of 19% (31–43%) for in-feed OGTs at 120 min [15] and 83–91% agreement between OST performed on different days [25], multiple factors can affect final test results. Furthermore, interpretation of OGT insulin concentrations should be accompanied by consideration of clinical findings when assessment of ID is used for diagnosing EMS or PPID related ID. Fluent transition from an insulin sensitive state to an insulin dysregulated state complicates the establishment of reliable cut-offs. However, it emphasizes the importance of early detection of horses being at high risk to develop metabolic pathologies and the importance of recording the degree of severity when individual therapy plans are created.

In conclusion, the standard dosed OGT with glucose application via naso-gastric tubing can be easily performed under clinical settings and allows reliable assessment of ID in horses.

Abbreviations
BW: bodyweight; CV: coefficient of variation; ELISA: enzyme-linked immunosorbent assay; EMS: equine metabolic syndrome; Fig: figure; ID: insulin dysregulation; IQR: interquartile range; IS: insulin sensitivity; OGT: oral glucose test; OST: oral sugar test; PPID: pituitary *pars intermedia* dysfunction; SVD: singular value decomposition.

Authors' contributions
TW and KF designed the study. TW and SS collected data. TW and JD analyzed data, wrote the manuscript and made figures. KH and KF helped to edit the manuscript. All authors read and approved the final manuscript.

Author details
[1] Clinic for Horses, University of Veterinary Medicine Hannover, Foundation, Bünteweg 9, 30559 Hannover, Germany. [2] Institute of Animal Science, Faculty of Agricultural Sciences, University of Hohenheim, Fruwirthstraße 35, 70593 Stuttgart, Germany.

Acknowledgements
The authors are grateful for technical support from Pia Schmidt during the sampling period and performance of the OGTs as well as Prof. Dr. W. Leibold for constructive cooperation.

Competing interests
The authors declare that they have no competing interests.

Availability of data and materials
The datasets used and/or analyzed during the current study are available from the corresponding author on reasonable request.

Consent for publication
Not applicable.

Ethics approval and consent to participate
Samples were collected during two studies which had been approved by the ethics committee within the University of Veterinary Medicine, Hannover, and the State Office for Consumer Protection and Food Safety in accordance with the German Animal Welfare Law (LAVES– Reference number: 33.14 42502-04-13/1259 and 33.12-42502-04-16/2341) as well as from insulin dysregulated horses and ponies during routine diagnostic procedures in the Clinic for Horses and owners provided informed consent that samples can be included in the study.

Funding
Parts of this research (LAVES– Reference number: 33.14 42502-04-13/1259) were financially supported by Boehringer-Ingelheim Vetmedica GmbH.

Publisher's Note
Springer Nature remains neutral with regard to jurisdictional claims in published maps and institutional affiliations.

Received: 22 October 2017   Accepted: 14 January 2018
Published online: 19 January 2018

References
1. Bertin FR, de Laat MA. The diagnosis of equine insulin dysregulation. Equine Vet J. 2017;49:570–6.
2. The Equine Endocrinology Group (EEG). Recommendations for the diagnosis and treatment of equine metabolic syndrome (EMS). https://sites.tufts.edu/equineendogroup/files/2016/11/2016-11-2-EMS-EEG-Final.pdf. Accessed 15 Dec 2016.
3. McFarlane D. Equine pituitary pars intermedia dysfunction. Vet Clin North Am Equine Pract. 2011;27:93–113.
4. The Equine Endocrinology Group (EEG). Recommendations for the diagnosis and treatment of pituitary pars intermedia dysfunction (PPID). 2015. https://sites.tufts.edu/equineendogroup/files/2015/12/2015-10-16_EEG-2015-recommendations.pdf. Accessed 15 Dec 2016.

MANUSCRIPT II

Warnken *et al. Acta Vet Scand (2018) 60:4*

Page 5 of 5

5. Pratt SE, Siciliano PD, Walston L. Variation of insulin sensitivity estimates in horses. J Equine Vet Sci. 2009;29:507–12.
6. Firshman AM, Valberg SJ. Factors affecting clinical assessment of insulin sensitivity in horses. Equine Vet J. 2007;39:567–75.
7. Frank N, Tadros EM. Insulin dysregulation. Equine Vet J. 2014;46:103–12.
8. Meier AD, de Laat MA, Reiche DB, Pollitt CC, Walsh DM, McGree JM, Sillence MN. The oral glucose test predicts laminitis risk in ponies fed a diet high in nonstructural carbohydrates. Domest Anim Endocrinol. 2018;63:1–9.
9. Smith S, Harris PA, Menzies-Gow NJ. Comparison of the in-feed glucose test and the oral sugar test. Equine Vet J. 2016;48:224–7.
10. Frank N, Geor R. Current best practice in clinical management of equine endocrine patients. Equine Vet Educ. 2014;26:6–9.
11. Schuver A, Frank N, Chameroy KA, Elliott SB. Assessment of insulin and glucose dynamics by using an oral sugar test in horses. J Equine Vet Sci. 2014;34:465–70.
12. Frank N. Equine metabolic syndrome. Vet Clin North Am Equine Pract. 2011;27:73–92.
13. Manfredi JM. Identifying breed differences in insulin dynamics, skeletal muscle and adipose tissue histology and biology. Dissertation, Michigan State University, 2016.
14. Lindase S, Nostell K, Brojer J. A modified oral sugar test for evaluation of insulin and glucose dynamics in horses. Acta Vet Scand. 2016;58(Suppl 1):64.
15. de Laat MA, Sillence MN. The repeatability of an oral glucose test in ponies. Equine Vet J. 2017;49:238–43.
16. Ralston SL. Insulin and glucose regulation. Vet Clin North Am Equine Pract. 2002;18:295–304.
17. Öberg J, Bröjer J, Wattle O, Lilliehöök I. Evaluation of an equine-optimized enzyme-linked immunosorbent assay for serum insulin measurement and stability study of equine serum insulin. Comp Clin Pathol. 2011;21:1291–300.
18. Warnken T, Huber K, Feige K. Comparison of three different methods for the quantification of equine insulin. BMC Vet Res. 2016;12:196.
19. Mercodia AB. Technical Note No: 34-0152: how to convert units when using Mercodia's animal insulin ELISAs. https://www.mercodia.com/assets/upload/files/TN34-0152%20converting%20insulin%20units%20v%201.pdf. Accessed 05 May 2017.
20. Fraley C, Raftery AE. Model-based clustering, discriminant analysis, and density estimation. J Am Stat Assoc. 2002;97:611–31.
21. Scrucca L, Raftery AE. Improved initialisation of model-based clustering using Gaussian hierarchical partitions. Adv Data Anal Classif. 2015;9:447–60.
22. Tinworth KD, Wynn PC, Boston RC, Harris PA, Sillence MN, Thevis M, Thomas A, Noble GK. Evaluation of commercially available assays for the measurement of equine insulin. Domest Anim Endocrinol. 2011;41:81–90.
23. Banse HE, McFarlane D. Comparison of three methods for evaluation of equine insulin regulation in horses of varied body condition score. J Equine Vet Sci. 2014;34:742–8.
24. Borer-Weir KE, Bailey SR, Menzies-Gow NJ, Harris PA, Elliott J. Evaluation of a commercially available radioimmunoassay and species-specific ELISAs for measurement of high concentrations of insulin in equine serum. Am J Vet Res. 2012;73:1596–602.
25. Frank N, Walsh DM. Repeatability of oral sugar test results, glucagon-like peptide-1 measurements, and serum high-molecular-weight adiponectin concentrations in horses. J Vet Intern Med. 2017;31:1178–87.

7 PART III – MANUSCRIPT III

Selection of assay used for insulin quantification impacts the results of oral glucose test and combined glucose-insulin test in horses

Tobias Warnken[1*], Marion Schmicke[2], Korinna Huber[3], Karsten Feige[1]

[1]   Clinic for Horses, University of Veterinary Medicine Hannover, Foundation,
       Bünteweg 9, 30559 Hannover, Germany

[2]   Clinic for Cattle, University of Veterinary Medicine Hannover, Foundation,
       Bischofsholer Damm 15, 30173 Hannover, Germany

          Current address: Institute of Agricultural and Nutritional Science,
          Faculty of Natural Sciences III, Martin-Luther-University Halle-
          Wittenberg, Theodor-Lieser-Straße 11, 06120 Halle (Saale), Germany

[3]   Institute of Animal Science, Faculty of Agricultural Sciences, University of
       Hohenheim, Fruwirthstraße 35, 70599 Stuttgart, Germany

*Corresponding author: Tobias Warnken

Prepared for submission.

Contribution to the manuscript

TW, KH and KF designed the study. TW collected and analyzed data, wrote
the manuscript and made figures. KH, MS and KF helped to edit the manuscript.
All authors read and approved the final manuscript.

Abstract

In clinical use, determination of disturbances in insulin regulation is part of the diagnostic procedure in horses and ponies suffering from metabolic pathologies such as the equine metabolic syndrome. Making a medical diagnosis requires exact quantification of equine insulin in serum or plasma. However, striking differences in absolute values obtained from different immunoassays exist. Most assays used in veterinary medicine include antibodies directed against human insulin, although amino acid sequences between equine and human insulin differ slightly. Therefore, the aim of this study was to compare results supplied by an equine-optimized insulin enzyme-linked immunosorbent assay (ELISA) and a frequently used immunoradiometric assay (IRMA) in samples obtained from two different diagnostic procedures. A total of 268 samples (oral glucose testing [OGT]: n = 117; combined glucose-insulin testing [CGIT]: n = 151) were used for the comparison of the two immunoassay methods. Samples were obtained from nine healthy horses during OGT and CGIT procedures. Insulin concentrations measured by ELISA and IRMA differed significantly ($p < 0.0001$) in samples from both diagnostic procedures. In addition to marked differences in absolute insulin concentrations between ELISA and IRMA, both methods showed a strong correlation when compared with OGT samples ($r = 0.97$; $p < 0.0001$) and CGIT samples ($r = 0.98$; $p < 0.0001$). Bland-Altman analysis indicated that the ELISA was an average of 40.94 ± 35.20 µIU/mL lower than the IRMA in samples obtained from the OGT procedure and even 90.82 ± 120 µIU/mL lower than the IRMA in samples obtained from the CGIT procedure, both with the presence of proportional error. Comparison of insulin curve progressions in OGT and CGIT differ significantly (OGT: $p < 0.0006$; CGIT: $p < 0.0002$) when insulin analyses were performed with ELISA or IRMA. These findings suggest that results between the assays should not be considered interchangeable. Moreover, insulin concentrations measured by different methods need to be interpreted carefully for making medical diagnosis, especially in clinically suspected cases where small changes in insulin levels can cause false classification of healthy or insulin-dysregulated horses in analyses of basal resting samples and samples from dynamic testing procedures.

Introduction

Insulin dysregulation (ID) is the key laboratory finding in horses and ponies suffering from equine metabolic syndrome (Durham et al. 2019). Based on poor sensitivity and the diagnostic value of resting or fasting, insulin concentrations for diagnosing ID dynamic testing protocols are currently recommended for a reliable assessment of impaired insulin regulation in horses and ponies (Frank et al. 2010, Frank 2011, Frank and Tadros 2014, Equine Endocrinology Group 2018, Durham et al. 2019). Veterinarians can choose between oral or intravenous test protocols, which reflect variable metabolic processes (Frank et al. 2010). Oral testing protocols, such as the oral glucose test (OGT), are simplified diagnostic procedures often used in clinical practice to assess ID in horses and ponies (Ralston 2002). Endogenous insulin response and blood glucose concentrations following orally administered glucose are determined for the diagnosis. Therefore, the OGT is considered as an indirect method to assess insulin sensitivity and focuses on the assessment of ID rather than specific tissue insulin resistance (IR). By contrast, the combined glucose insulin test (CGIT) is considered to be a direct method to assess tissue insulin sensitivity and IR and is based on the injection of insulin and glucose followed by measurements of the plasma disappearance of both (Eiler et al. 2005). In contrast to the OGT, the CGIT only tests the capacity of the exogenous insulin to shift the injected glucose into insulin-sensitive tissues. In addition to the differences in the underlying physiological backgrounds of both tests, the exact quantification of insulin by laboratory analysis is the most important and challenging step to diagnose changes in insulin regulation. Veterinary diagnostic laboratories use different assays for the quantification of equine insulin and several studies have highlighted differences between assays and revealed significant discrepancies between frequently used methods for quantification of equine insulin in research and clinical settings (Öberg et al. 2011, Tinworth et al. 2011, Borer-Weir et al. 2012b, Banse et al. 2014, Warnken et al. 2016, Carslake et al. 2017). No assay with a specific antibody directed against equine insulin is available. Thus, there was a need for alternatives. Therefore, several immunoassays previously designed for analyses of human or laboratory animal insulin were used in veterinary laboratories. Most commercial immunoassays are based on antibodies directed against human or non-equine insulin. Moreover, several previous studies and established reference ranges and cutoff values for diagnostic procedures are based on results obtained by use of a human-specific insulin radioimmunoassay (RIA) (Coat-a-Count Insulin RIA, Siemens Medical Solutions Diagnostics, Los Angeles, CA, USA) previously being extensively validated for the use in equids (Eiler et al. 2005, Frank et al. 2006, Frank et al. 2010). However, an evaluation of insulin assays for replacement and clinical applicability was necessary due to the current unavailability of the assay. Therefore, the aim of our study was to compare insulin concentrations supplied by a immunoradiometric assay (IRMA) (Insulin(e) IRMA KIT, Beckman Coulter, Prague, Czech Republic) with results obtained from an equine-optimized ELISA (Equine Insulin ELISA, Mercodia AB, Uppsala, Sweden) in serum samples obtained during OGT and CGIT procedures in consideration of the presence of endogenous equine insulin during OGT and mainly exogenous non-equine insulin in CGIT procedures.

Materials and Methods

Animals and samples

Nine healthy warmblood breed horses of unknown insulin sensitivity were included in the study. There were five mares, two geldings and two stallions, aged (mean±SD) 16±7.8 years, weighed 539±68 kg, with mean body condition score (BCS) of 4.2±1.4. Horses underwent dynamic diagnostic testing for evaluation of insulin dysregulation with oral glucose test (OGT) and for tissue insulin resistance with combined glucose insulin test (CGIT). For implementation of OGT 1 g/kg BW glucose powder (Glukose, WDT, Garbsen, Germany) dissolved in two liters water was administered by naso-gastric tubing (Ralston 2002). Blood samples were collected via jugular vein catheter (EquiCathTM Fastflow, Braun Vet Care GmbH, Germany) for a three-hour period. For implementation of the CGIT two intravenous indwelling catheters (EquiCathTM Fastflow, Braun Vet Care GmbH, Germany) were aseptically implanted in each jugular vein of the horses. One catheter was used for administration of glucose solution and insulin, whereas the second one was used for the collection of blood samples for three hours. To carry out the CGIT, 150 mg/kg BW glucose solution

(Glucose 500 mg/mL, B. Braun Melsungen AG, Germany) were injected intravenously as a bolus within 1 minute, immediately followed by 0.1 IU/kg BW porcine zinc-insulin (Caninsulin® 40 I.E./ml, MSD, Unterschleißheim, Germany) and 20 ml saline solution (NaCl; 0,9 %; B. Braun Melsungen AG, Germany) to flush the catheter. Blood samples were placed into plain tubes for serum preparation and centrifuged after 60 minutes incubation at room temperature at 1000 g for 6 minutes. Thereafter, samples were aliquoted and stored at 80°C until further analysis. In total 117 serum samples from OGT procedure and 151 serum samples from CGIT procedure were available and used for comparison of insulin concentrations measured by ELISA and IRMA.

Insulin analyses

Serum insulin concentrations were analyzed by use of a human-specific RIA (Insulin(e) IRMA KIT, Beckman Coulter, Prague, Czech Republic) and by use of an equine-optimized insulin ELISA (Equine Insulin ELISA, Mercodia AB, Uppsala, Sweden). The equine-optimized insulin assay is a solid phase two-side sandwich ELISA for the quantification of equine insulin in serum or plasma. It is based on monoclonal mouse anti-porcine insulin antibodies coupled to plate and free monoclonal mouse anti-porcine insulin antibodies labeled with horseradish peroxidase. Samples were processed prior to change of standards in the assay from µg/L to µIU/mL. The limit of detection for this assay is 0.01 µg/L, specificity of the assay is stated at 100 % for porcine insulin and cross-reactivity with human insulin is 22 % (according to the manufacturer's protocol). Samples with insulin concentrations greater than the highest value of the standard curve (>1.5 µg/L; corresponding range in µIU/mL: >172.5) were diluted with assay specific sample buffer (Diabetes Sample Buffer, Mercodia AB, Uppsala, Sweden). Samples were analyzed in duplicates.

Coincidently, OGT and CGIT serum samples were analyzed for insulin by the human-specific radioimmunoassay (Insulin(e) IRMA KIT, Beckman Coulter, Prague, Czech Republic), which is often used for analyses of insulin in various animal species (Muscher-Banse et al. 2012, Locher et al. 2015, Schulz et al. 2015, Kinoshita et al. 2016). This assay uses sandwich technique and is based on mouse monoclonal antibodies directed against two different epitopes of insulin. The first antibody is coated to the tubes and the second one is labelled with iodine125. The stated limit of detection is 2.9 µIU/mL. The corresponding measurement ranges extends from 2.9 to 300 µIU/mL. No information about cross-reactivity for equine or animal insulin is given by the manufacturer. The calibrators used in this RIA were calibrated against the international standard WHO 1st IRP 66/304. Samples with insulin concentrations greater than the highest value of the standard curve were diluted with assay buffer.

Table 1: Information about the insulin assays

Assay	Standards	Primary antibody	Secondary antibody
Mercodia Equine Insulin ELISA	porcine insulin	mouse monoclonal anti-porcine insulin	mouse monoclonal anti-porcine insulin HRP-conjugate
Beckman Coulter Insulin(e) IRMA KIT	human recombinant insulin	mouse monoclonal anti-insulin	mouse monoclonal anti-insulin labelled with iodine [125]

Data analyses and statistics

Data supplied by the ELISA had to be converted from "µg/L" into the commonly used unit "µIU/mL" to compare the insulin concentrations obtained between assays and results reported in previous studies. The manufacturer of the ELISA offered a specific conversion factor (1 µg/L = 115 mU/L) for the conversion of data supplied by the equine-optimized insulin ELISA from µg/L to µIU/mL (Ab 2017) which was used for the calculation of data in our study. Data analysis was performed using GraphPad Prism software (version 7.02; GraphPad Inc. La Jolla, CA, USA). Data were tested for normality using the Shapiro-Wilk normality test. Wilcoxon signed rank test, Spearman correlation and Deming regression analyses were used to compare results from different assays as a whole and at specific time points and to evaluate relationships between both methods. Bland-Altman analysis was performed to calculate the method-dependent bias and 95 % limits of agreement between both methods. Repeated measures two-way ANOVA with Sidak's multiple comparisons test was performed to compare results supplied by IRMA and ELISA in OGT and

CGIT over the testing period. Statistical significance was accepted when p < 0.05. All values are expressed as mean ± SD unless otherwise indicate.

Results

Assay performance data

Equine-optimized ELISA

Intra-assay CV was 4.61 % at low equine insulin concentrations (2.34 µIU/mL) and 1.91 % at high insulin concentrations (108.81 µIU/mL). Inter-assay CV was 5.27 %, 3.24 % and 3.17 % for low, medium and high commercial animal insulin controls, respectively. Inter-assay CV for equine serum samples were 7.43 % and 4.83 % for low (10.53 µIU/mL) and high (109.98 µIU/mL) insulin concentrations, respectively. The linearity of dilution was indicated by linear regression with r2 = 0.9994 and p < 0.0001 and recovery upon dilution was 95.9 ± 4.6 %.

Human-specific IRMA

Intra-assay CV was 8.2 % at medium equine insulin concentrations (32.4 µIU/mL) and 11.5 % at high insulin concentrations (120.5 µIU/mL). Inter-assay CV was 9.4 % for medium and 12.5 % for high equine insulin concentrations. Inter-assay CV was 6.5 % for low and 8.4 % for high commercial assay controls. The linearity of dilution was indicated by linear regression with r2 = 0.9995 and p < 0.0001 and recovery upon dilution was 97.3 ± 4.8 %.

Samples from OGT

Insulin concentrations measured in OGT samples ranged from 2.98 to 125.4 µIU/mL in ELISA analyses and from 4.42 to 275.0 µIU/mL in RIA analyses (Figure 1a). OGT samples' insulin concentrations measured with the ELISA were significantly (p < 0.0001) lower than insulin concentrations measured with the IRMA (Figure 1a). The ELISA and IRMA insulin concentrations were significantly correlated (r = 0.97; p < 0.0001) (Figure 2a). Deming regression analysis is shown in Figure 2a. Bland-Altman plot analysis for ELISA minus IRMA in OGT samples revealed a bias of -40.94 ± 35.20 µIU/ml and 95 % limits of agreement from -109.9 to 28.06 µIU/mL (Figure 3a). Basal insulin concentrations prior to OGT and insulin concentrations after 120 min during OGT determined by both assays differed significantly ($p < 0.0008$; $p > 0.0024$, respectively) when compared by Wilcoxon matched-pairs signed rank test. Statistical analysis with RM two-way ANOVA indicated significant differences for the factor time ($p < 0.0001$) and analysis method ($p = 0.0006$) and an interaction of both ($p < 0.0001$) in the OGT procedure. Insulin concentrations differ significantly from time point 45 min until the end of the sampling period between both methods (Figure 4a).

Samples from CGIT

Insulin concentrations in CGIT samples ranged from 2.47 to 640.4 µIU/mL in ELISA analyses and from 5.21 to 1124.0 µIU/mL in IRMA analyses (Figure 1b). Insulin concentrations of CGIT samples measured with the ELISA were significantly ($p < 0.0001$) lower than insulin concentrations measured with the IRMA (Figure 1b). Spearman correlation with both methods revealed good correlation ($r = 0.9799$; $p < 0.0001$) for CGIT samples and Deming regression analysis is shown in Figure 2b. Bland-Altman analysis for ELISA minus IRMA in CGIT samples revealed a bias of -90.82 ± 128.0 µIU/ml and 95 % limits of agreement from -341.7 to 160.1 µIU/mL (Figure 3b). Basal endogenous insulin concentrations prior to CGIT and insulin concentrations after 45 min during CGIT containing mainly exogenous insulin determined by both assays differed significantly ($p < 0.0034$; $p < 0.0078$) when compared by Wilcoxon matched-pairs signed rank test. Equal to the situation in OGT samples' analyses, the RM two-way ANOVA in the CGIT procedure indicated significant differences for the factor time ($p < 0.0001$) and analysis method ($p = 0.0002$) and an interaction ($p < 0.0001$). Insulin concentrations differ significantly from time point 3 min until 15 min between both methods (Figure 4b), where relatively high concentrations were measured with both methods.

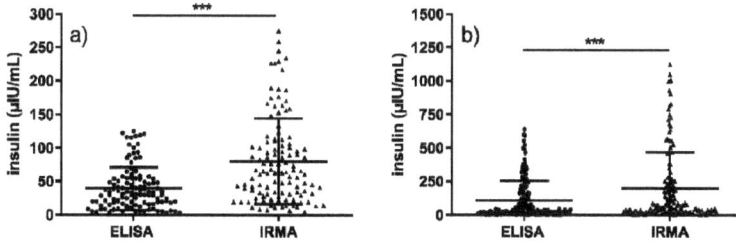

Figure 1: Insulin concentrations measured in samples obtained during a) oral glucose testing procedure (OGT; n=117) and b) combined glucose-insulin testing procedure (CGIT; n=151) with ELISA and IRMA. Data were analyzed by Wilcoxon matched-pairs rank test. *** p < 0.001.

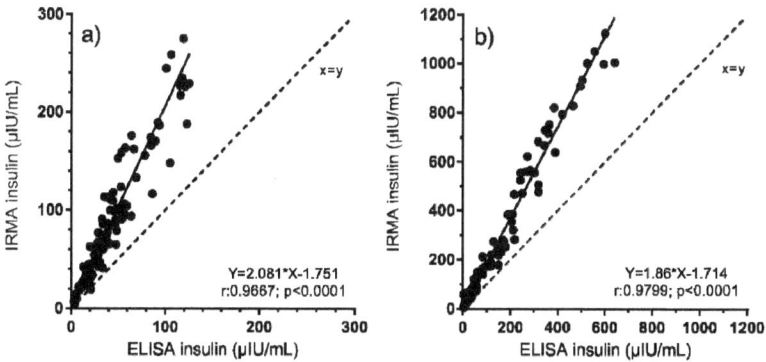

Figure 2: Scatterplot of measurement results for a) OGT samples (n=117) and b) CGIT samples (n=151) from ELISA analyses compared to IRMA analyses.

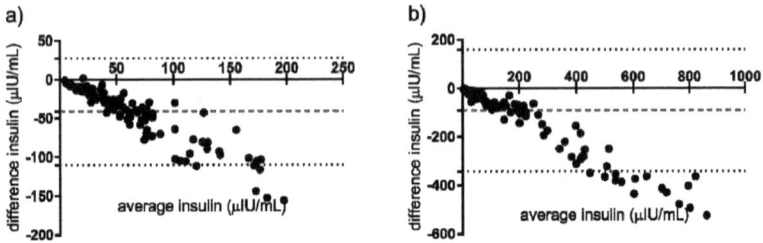

Figure 3: Bland-Altman plot of average compared to difference ELISA minus IRMA in a) OGT samples (n = 117), b) CGIT samples (n = 151). Dashed line = bias, pointed line = 95 % limits of agreements.

Discussion

Clinical diagnosis of ID or IR in horses with suspected equine metabolic syndrome or other neuroendocrine diseases such as PPID is based on the assessment of the insulinemic state of the horse or pony (Durham et al. 2019). Reliable quantification of insulin is required for safe and accurate diagnosis. Results of the present study indicated marked differences in insulin concentrations derived from measures with the equine-optimized ELISA and the human-specific IRMA. Differences also occurred in samples collected during both diagnostic procedures, OGT and CGIT. Consequently, method-specific variations in insulin concentrations influence clinical interpretation concerning the patient's insulinemic state. Nevertheless, both methods were able to detect the increase and decrease in insulin concentrations during dynamic diagnostic testing procedure. Furthermore, low, moderate and high insulin concentrations, although on different concentration levels, could be differentiated by both assays.

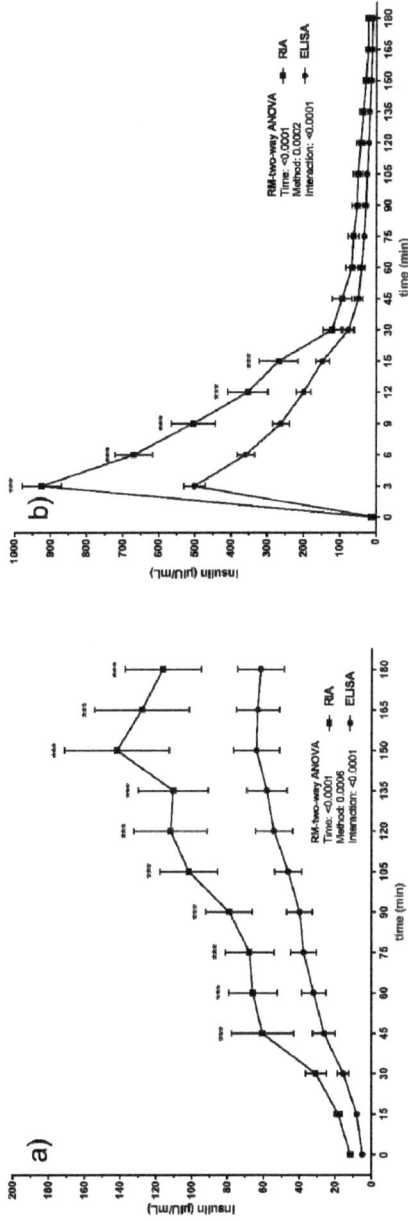

Figure 4: Insulin concentrations during a) OGT and b) CGIT procedure measured with ELISA and IRMA. RM-two-way ANOVA and Sidak's multiple comparisons test. *** p < 0.001.

Analyses of insulin in basal or resting samples

Measures of basal or resting insulin concentrations have often been used to identify insulin dysregulated equids due to the simplicity of the procedure. Therefore, correct analyses of low to moderate insulin concentrations is as important as correct analyses of high insulin concentrations after stimulation. Basal insulin concentrations were significantly higher in IRMA compared to the ELISA. Interestingly, analyses of fasted basal samples with the ELISA investigated resulted even in markedly higher insulin concentrations compared to a commonly used chemiluminescence assay (CLIA) (ADVIA Centaur Insulin Assay, Siemens Healthcare Diagnostics GmbH, Eschborn, Germany) in a previous study (Warnken et al. 2016). Thus, the concentrations supplied by the human-specific IRMA also seem to be significantly higher compared to the CLIA mentioned previously.

Furthermore, Banse et al. (2014) compared the previously well validated and used human-specific RIA (Coat-a-Count Insulin RIA, Siemens Medical Solutions Diagnostics, Los Angeles, CA, USA) with another commercially available CLIA (IMMULITE 1000 Insulin Assay, Siemens Healthcare Diagnostics, Tarrytown, NY, USA). Analyses of serum samples of 40 horses covered a broad range of insulin concentrations; however, poor recovery rates for samples spiked with an equine insulin standard (Equine Insulin Standard, Shibayagi Co., Ishihara, Japan) and poor accordance between both methods were reported (Banse et al. 2014). These findings further complicate the clinical interpretation in the context of reference ranges and cutoff values for basal insulin concentrations defined previously. Koeller et al. (2016) reported a reference range of 2.0 to 21.1 µIU/mL based on analyses with the a human-specific CLIA (IMMULITE 2000, Siemens Healthcare Diagnostics, Eschborn, Germany), whereas the most cited and clinically widely used reference for basal insulin concentrations of > 20 µIU/mL was calculated based on analyses with human-specific RIA (Coat-a-Count RIA, Diagnostic Products Corporation, Los Angeles, California, USA) (Treiber et al. 2006, Carter et al. 2009). This might be in contrast to Carslake et al. (2017) reporting that the same CLIA (IMMULITE 2000, Siemens Healthcare Diagnostics, Camberley, Surrey, UK) tends to provide lower insulin concentrations than the RIA (Coat-a-Count RIA, Diagnostic Products

Corporation, Los Angeles, California, USA) in the analytical range of the reported cutoff values for basal insulin. These findings highlighted the importance of the consideration of the immunoassay used for analyses of insulin concentrations in the patient samples.

Analyzes of insulin in oral glycemic challenges

Depending on the testing protocol, glucose application route, glucose dosage and sampling time point, multiple cutoff values are described in literature to distinguish between healthy and diseased horses (Ralston 2002, Schuver et al. 2014, Smith et al. 2016, Warnken et al. 2018). However, these studies used varying immunoassay methods for the quantification of insulin and diverse test protocols. Therefore, these cutoff values or reference ranges are only applicable in a combination with the individual testing protocol and the specific immunoassay used. If insulin concentrations at 120 min during OGT in the present study were interpreted regardless of the analysis method based on a previously defined cutoff value of 110 µlU/mL (Warnken et al. 2018), the ELISA analysis indicated 1/9 horses as ID, whereas IRMA analyses indicated 5/9. Differences in insulin concentrations in samples obtained during glucose tolerance testing analyzed by another human-specific RIA (Coat-a-Count Insulin RIA, Siemens Medical Solutions Diagnostics, Los Angeles, CA, USA) and the equine-optimized insulin ELISA used in the present study have been described (Tinworth et al. 2011). In this study, the equine-optimized ELISA revealed significantly lower insulin concentrations in 17/18 samples compared to the human-specific RIA, while 1/18 samples were measured higher in the ELISA compared to the RIA. In the same study, six assays were investigated in terms of performance and only the equine-optimized ELISA passed the requested standards for precision, accuracy and specificity straightaway. However, compared to liquid chromatography and high-resolution/high-accuracy mass spectrometry (LC-MS), the equine-optimized ELISA and the human-specific RIA underestimated the equine insulin concentrations, with the ELISA being even worse (Tinworth et al. 2011). Thus, the authors concluded that both assays were not able to detect endogenous equine insulin satisfactorily when the LC-MS technique is considered as a gold standard. However, the samples used have been preprocessed by use of a catching step with anti-insulin antibodies prior to LC-MS analyses. In addition, insulin-aspart, a fast-acting recombinant insulin analogue, was used as the internal standard. Taken together, both procedures challenge the actual significance of these results.

In addition to a good correlation between ELISA and IRMA in the present study, results from Bland-Altman plot analysis revealed the importance of proportional error between both methods, indicating that the difference between both methods was even exacerbated with an increased insulin concentration. This situation precluded simplified conversion. Taking into account that only healthy animals were used in this study, this bias may even be amplified when samples from clinically affected insulin-dysregulated patients were analyzed with even higher insulin responses in the OGT procedure. Analysis with the IRMA generally supplied consistently higher insulin concentrations for the identical sample compared to the ELISA analysis in this study. Differences between both methods may be explained by differences in the underlying antibodies of the assays. The IRMA is based on monoclonal anti-human insulin antibodies, whereas the ELISA is based on monoclonal anti-porcine insulin antibodies. The equine insulin molecule has more similarity in the amino acid sequence with the porcine insulin molecule (the only difference is in the A-chain at position 9) than with the human insulin molecule (two different amino acids at position 9 in the A-chain and position 30 in the B-chain) (Ho et al. 2008, Kuuranne et al. 2008). Therefore, it was expected that the equine-optimized porcine-specific insulin ELISA would supply more exact concentrations compared to the IRMA based on antibodies directed against human insulin. Although the IRMA is based on antibodies directed against a molecule with less similarity in the amino acid sequence, it revealed higher concentrations compared to the ELISA. Since sample analysis with LC-MS is lacking and the equine insulin standard was not available at the time the study was performed, it could not be stated whether the IRMA overestimated or the ELISA underestimated the real sample insulin concentration.

Analytical ranges, impact of dilution and clinical consequences

High insulin concentrations might occur in samples obtained during the OGT procedure when patients suffer from severe ID. Measuring ranges of the assay are limited but are expected to be reliable for low and high insulin concentrations in samples received for analyses obtained during dynamic diagnostic tests. The measurement range for the IRMA is 0.49 to 300 µIU/mL. Regarding the sensitivity, it is important to mention that the analytical sensitivity of 0.49 µIU/mL is in contrast to the functional sensitivity of 1.35 µIU/mL. The IRMA provides a wider range compared to the equine-optimized ELISA with a measurement range from 0.02 to 1.5 µg/L corresponding to 2.3 to 172.5 µIU/mL and an analytical sensitivity of 0.01 µg/L (1.15 µIU/mL). Based on this, expanding the range by sample dilution might be necessary in some cases. Whereas the samples obtained during the OGT procedure in the present study were all measured undiluted within the measurement range of the assay, samples obtained during the CGIT procedure were diluted prior to analyses in both assays due to expected high initial insulin concentrations. Based on the excellent RUD and dilution parallelism, the results can be considered as valid concentrations. Nevertheless, dilution often impairs results when performed with the dilution medium provided by the manufacturer (Tinworth et al. 2011, Carslake et al. 2017). Both studies reported a significant improvement of dilution if charcoal-stripped serum was used. Based on these difficulties resulting from dilution, most laboratories do not report insulin concentrations above the upper range of the analytical range. However, there is growing evidence to support the hypothesis that high insulin concentrations are associated with more severe lameness in laminitis cases (De Laat et al. 2019) or risk of laminitis in cases with severe ID (Meier et al. 2017), thus, highlighting the clinical relevance and importance of reporting absolute values in samples containing high insulin concentrations.

Analyzes of insulin concentrations in intravenous challenges with presence of exogenous insulin

Human recombinant insulin is recommended for implementation of CGIT developed by Eiler et al. (2005). The diagnosis of IR during CGIT is mainly based on the assessment of the insulin-mediated glucose kinetics and, additionally, on the clearance of the applied exogenous insulin from plasma within 45 min. It is important to mention that the quantification of insulin in blood samples obtained during some IV tests can lead to potential cross-reactivity due to the presence of endogenous equine insulin and exogenous injected human insulin or other non-equine insulin analogues. Therefore, selection of an appropriate assay is necessary. Ideally, sample cross-analysis with a human-specific and an equine-specific method is needed to allow the exact assessment regarding differentiation between both. In the above mentioned publication, blood samples were analyzed by use of the human-specific RIA (Coat-A-Count RIA, Diagnostic Products Corp, Los Angeles, California, USA) (Eiler et al. 2005), thus, expecting the assay to detect 100 % of the recombinant human insulin based on the assays underlying anti-human insulin antibodies. The recombinant human insulin formulation used originally is not composed of substitutions of amino acids at various positions to impair pharmacokinetics towards short- or long-acting properties. Insulin analogues are characterized by substitutions at various amino acids or additions of residues to the COOH terminus of the B chain for impairment of their pharmacokinetics for special issues (Standel 2002). If a CGIT is performed, one should be aware that, firstly, the insulin analogue used may alter test results and, secondly, the impaired pharmacokinetics of the insulin analogues may impact the glucose and insulin kinetics (Warnken 2018). Several insulin analogues have been investigated in human medicine for cross-reactivity, because alterations due to cross-reactivity between endogenous human insulin and injected insulin analogues are a common problem in insulin analysis if patients are treated for diabetes type 1 (Owen and Roberts 2004, Dayaldasani et al. 2015). Some of the immunoassay methods investigated have also been frequently used in veterinary medicine (IMMULITE® systems and ADVIA Centaur XP systems both from Siemens Healthcare Diagnostics). Depending on the insulin analog selected, the ADVIA Centaur XP revealed cross-reactivity in human samples with insulin analogues of up to 152 % (Owen and Roberts 2004), whereas the IMMULITE 2000 revealed less cross-reactivity of up to 42 %. This questions what would be measured in samples obtained from CGITs and analyzed with these assays. However, the CGITs carried out in the present study were implemented by injection of porcine-zinc insulin. As mentioned earlier, the porcine insulin molecule and the equine insulin molecule only differ in one amino acid at position A9, whereas human insulin molecule differs from equine insulin molecule at position A9 and position B30 (Ho et al. 2008). Position B30 is considered important for the tertiary structure of the protein and can impair sufficient formation of antigen-antibody complexes, which is essential for analyses with immunoassays (Conlon 2001, Kuuranne et al. 2008). It was expected that the porcine insulin molecule could act in a more comparable fashion to the physiological endogenous equine insulin and that laboratory analyses with the equine-optimized insulin ELISA based on mouse monoclonal anti-porcine insulin antibodies could allow exact quantification of endogenous equine insulin and applied exogenous porcine zinc insulin in a CGIT procedure (cross-reactivity 100 % according to the manufacturer). By contrast, sample analyses with the human-specific insulin IRMA was suspected of supplying an impaired insulin concentration due to insufficient antigen-antibody binding caused by the underlying mouse monoclonal antibodies directed against two different epitopes of the human insulin molecule. Interestingly, again, the IRMA supplied the significantly and consistently higher insulin concentrations compared to the ELISA when samples from the CGIT procedure were compared. A potential explanation might be that, despite the general higher level of supplied insulin concentrations by the IRMA, the responsible binding epitope of the antibodies used in the IRMA binds to a region of the amino acid sequence of the insulin molecule which is similar between equids and humans, hence, allowing unimpaired detection. However, differences between both analyses exist and whereas ELISA analyses supplied insulin concentrations above 100 µIU/mL after 45 min in 1/9 horses, IRMA analyses supplied 2/9, again causing different classification and incorrect diagnosis of IR based on the interpretation of the insulin concentration during testing. It is important to point out that no study is available redefining the 45-min insulin cutoff value with currently available methods used for the quantification of equine insulin. In general, for insulin analyses in samples obtained during a regular CGIT or even hyperinsulinemic euglycemic clamp procedure with regular human recombinant insulin, laboratory methods based on human-specific anti-insulin antibodies might provide advantages compared to porcine- or equine-specific assays. Thus, it is important to be aware of the analyte of interest, which could be the endogenous equine insulin in oral glycemic tests or the non-equine insulin in several IV tests when choosing the immunoassay for sample analyses. Therefore, samples might be processed with different immunoassays focusing on either human or non-equine insulin with respect to the potential cross-reactivity by the different assays as like for example performed by Lindase et al. (2017).

Some immunoassay comparisons or validation studies have been performed with sample material obtained during oral glycemic challenges, during IV challenge tests (Borer-Weir et al. 2012a) or even via hyperinsulinemic glycemic clamp studies (Carslake et al. 2017), thus, using samples with a mixture of endogenous equine and exogenous non-equine insulin for the evaluation of the assay performance in terms of equine-specificity. Despite the fact that the insulin analogues used for the IV testing procedure were not stated, regular human insulin was probably used. Keeping this in mind, at least part of the missing or striking accordance reported between different immunoassay investigated should be interpreted with care and need attention based on the potential presence off cross-reactivity, which might contribute to the variable outcome of sample analyses with the different immunoassays.

In conclusion, insulin measurements after OGT and CGIT differ significantly depending on the choice of immunoassay. These findings suggest that results between the assays should not be considered interchangeable. Thus, the diagnosis of ID assessed by OGT or of IR assessed by CGIT requires consideration of the immunoassay used for the quantification of insulin. The presence especially of exogenous insulin in samples obtained from IV testing for the assessment of IR might contribute to variable outcome due to potential cross-reactivity of the exogenous insulin molecules or analogues with the assay antibodies. Furthermore, assessment of the management and therapy success or re-assessment of patients requires the use of the same laboratory and the same assay for the interpretation of results over time.

References

Banse H. E., Mccann J., Yang F., Wagg C. and Mcfarlane D. (2014) Comparison of two methods for measurement of equine insulin. J Vet Diagn Invest, 4, 527–530

Borer-Weir K. E., Bailey S. R., Menzies-Gow N. J., Harris P. A. and Elliott J. (2012) Evaluation of a commercially available radioimmunoassay and species-specific ELISAs for measurement of high concentrations of insulin in equine serum. Am J Vet Res, 10, 1596–1602

Carslake H. B., Pinchbeck G. L. and Mcgowan C. M. (2017) Evaluation of a Chemiluminescent Immunoassay for Measurement of Equine Insulin. J Vet Intern Med, 2, 568–574

Carter R. A., Treiber K. H., Geor R. J., Douglass L. and Harris P. A. (2009) Prediction of incipient pasture-associated laminitis from hyperinsulinaemia, hyperleptinaemia and generalised and localised obesity in a cohort of ponies. Equine Vet J, 2, 171–178

Conlon J. M. (2001) Evolution of the insulin molecule: insights into structure-activity and phylogenetic relationships. Peptides, 7, 1183–1193

Dayaldasani A., Rodríguez Espinosa M., Ocón Sánchez P. and Pérez Valero V. (2015) Cross-reactivity of insulin analogues with three insulin assays. Ann Clin Biochem, 3, 312–318

De Laat M. A., Sillence M. N. and Reiche D. B. (2019) Phenotypic, hormonal, and clinical characteristics of equine endocrinopathic laminitis. J Vet Intern Med, 3, 1456–1463

Durham A. E., Frank N., McGowan C. M., Menzies-Gow N. J., Roelfsema E., Vervuert I., Feige K. and Fey K. (2019) ECEIM consensus statement on equine metabolic syndrome. J Vet Intern Med, 2, 335–349

Eiler H., Frank N., Andrews F. M., Oliver J. W. and Fecteau K. A. (2005) Physiologic assessment of blood glucose homeostasis via combined intravenous glucose and insulin testing in horses. Am J Vet Res, 9, 1598–1604

Equine Endocrinology Group – Frank N., Bailey S., Bertin F. R., Burns T., De Laat M., Durham A., Kritchevsky J., Menzies-Gow N., Tadros L. (2018) Recommendations for the diagnosis and treatment of Equine Metabolic Syndrome (EMS). https://sites.tufts.edu/equineendogroup/files/2018/09/2018-Final-EMS_Recommendations_Web.pdf. Accessed 05 Nov 2018.

Equine Endocrinology Group – Schott H., Andrews F., Durham A., Frank N., Hart K., Kritchevsky J., McFarlane D., Tadros L. (2017) Recommendations for the Diagnosis and Treatment of Pituitary Pars Intermedia Dysfunction (PPID). https://sites.tufts.edu/equineendogroup/files/2017/11/2017-EEG-Recommendations-PPID.pdf. Accessed 12 Nov 2018.

Frank N. (2011) Equine metabolic syndrome. Vet Clin North Am Equine Pract, 1, 73–92

Frank N., Elliott S. B., Brandt L. E. and Keisler D. H. (2006) Physical characteristics, blood hormone concentrations, and plasma lipid concentrations in obese horses with insulin resistance. J Am Vet Med Assoc, 9, 1383–1390

Frank N., Geor R. J., Bailey S. R., Durham A. E., Johnson P. J. and American College of Veterinary Internal M. (2010) Equine metabolic syndrome. J Vet Intern Med, 3, 467–475

Frank N. and Tadros E. M. (2014) Insulin dysregulation. Equine Vet J, 1, 103–112

Ho E. N., Wan T. S., Wong A. S., Lam K. K. and Stewart B. D. (2008) Doping control analysis of insulin and its analogues in equine plasma by liquid chromatography-tandem mass spectrometry. J Chromatogr A, 2, 183–190

Kinoshita A., Kenez A., Locher L., Meyer U., Danicke S., Rehage J. and Huber K. (2016) Insulin Signaling in Liver and Adipose Tissues in Periparturient Dairy Cows Supplemented with Dietary Nicotinic Acid. PLoS One, 1, e0147028

Koeller G., Bassewitz K. and Schusser G. F. (2016) Reference ranges of insulin, insulin like growth factor-1 and adrenocorticotropic hormone in ponies. Tierarztl Prax Ausg G Grosstiere Nutztiere, 1, 19–25

Kuuranne T., Thomas A., Leinonen A., Delahaut P., Bosseloir A., Schanzer W. and Thevis M. (2008) Insulins in equine urine: qualitative analysis by immunoaffinity purification and liquid chromatography/tandem mass spectrometry for doping control purposes in horse-racing. Rapid Commun Mass Spectrom, 3, 355–362

Lindase S., Nostell K., Soder J. and Brojer J. (2017) Relationship Between beta-cell Response and Insulin Sensitivity in Horses based on the Oral Sugar Test and the Euglycemic Hyperinsulinemic Clamp. J Vet Intern Med, 5, 1541–1550

Locher L., Haussler S., Laubenthal L., Singh S. P., Winkler J., Kinoshita A., Kenez A., Rehage J., Huber K., Sauerwein H. and Danicke S. (2015) Effect of increasing body condition on key regulators of fat metabolism in subcutaneous adipose tissue depot and circulation of nonlactating dairy cows. J Dairy Sci, 2, 1057–1068

Meier A. D., De Laat M. A., Reiche D. B., Pollitt C. C., Walsh D. M., Mcgree J. M. and Sillence M. N. (2017) The oral glucose test predicts laminitis risk in ponies fed a diet high in nonstructural carbohydrates. Domest Anim Endocrinol, 63, 1–9

Muscher-Banse A. S., Piechotta M., Schroder B. and Breves G. (2012) Modulation of intestinal glucose transport in response to reduced nitrogen supply in young goats. J Anim Sci, 13, 4995–5004

Öberg J., Bröjer J., Wattle O. and Lilliehöök I. (2011) Evaluation of an equine-optimized enzyme-linked immunosorbent assay for serum insulin measurement and stability study of equine serum insulin. Comp Clin Path, 6, 1291–1300

Owen W. E. and Roberts W. L. (2004) Cross-Reactivity of Three Recombinant Insulin Analogs with Five Commercial Insulin Immunoassays. Clin Chem, 1, 257–259

Ralston S. L. (2002) Insulin and glucose regulation. Vet Clin North Am Equine Pract, 2, 295–304

Schulz K., Frahm J., Kersten S., Meyer U., Rehage J., Piechotta M., Meyerholz M., Breves G., Reiche D., Sauerwein H. and Dänicke S. (2015) Effects of Inhibiting Dipeptidyl Peptidase-4 (DPP4) in Cows with Subclinical Ketosis. PLOS ONE, 8, e0136078

Schuver A., Frank N., Chameroy K. A. and Elliott S. B. (2014) Assessment of Insulin and Glucose Dynamics by Using an Oral Sugar Test in Horses. J Equine Vet Sci, 4, 465–470

Smith S., Harris P. A. and Menzies-Gow N. J. (2016) Comparison of the in-feed glucose test and the oral sugar test. Equine Vet J, 2, 224–227

Standl E. (2002) Insulin analogues – State of the art. Horm Res, 57 Suppl 1, 40–5

Tinworth K. D., Wynn P. C., Boston R. C., Harris P. A., Sillence M. N., Thevis M., Thomas A. and Noble G. K. (2011) Evaluation of commercially available assays for the measurement of equine insulin. Domest Anim Endocrinol, 2, 81–90

Treiber K. H., Kronfeld D. S., Hess T. M., Byrd B. M., Splan R. K. and Staniar W. B. (2006) Evaluation of genetic and metabolic predispositions and nutritional risk factors for pasture-associated laminitis in ponies. J Am Vet Med Assoc, 10, 1538–1545

Warnken T., Delarocque J., Schumacher S., Huber K. and Feige K. (2018) Retrospective analysis of insulin responses to standard dosed oral glucose tests

(OGTs) via naso-gastric tubing towards definition of an objective cut-off value. Acta Vet Scand, 1, 4

Warnken T., Huber K. and Feige K. (2016) Comparison of three different methods for the quantification of equine insulin. BMC Vet Res, 1, 196

Warnken T., Reiche D., Huber K., Feige K. (2018) Comparison of endocrine and metabolic responses to oral glucose test and combined glucose-insulin tests in horses. Pferdeheilkunde, 34, 316–326

8 GENERAL DISCUSSION

Equine metabolic syndrome is an increasing problem and health concern in the equine population. Recent research suggests that hyperinsulinemia is the only one among the cluster of signs and symptoms that characterize EMS that is clearly linked to the development of laminitis (Durham et al. 2019). The prevalence of hyperinsulinemia reflecting ID as the central key factor of EMS has been reported in publications with 18 to 27 % of horses and ponies being hyperinsulinemic (Pleasant et al. 2013; Morgan et al. 2014). However, cases presented to a first opinion hospital for evaluation of laminitis have been hyperinsulinemic in 66 % of the cases (Karikoski et al. 2011), highlighting the clinical relevance of endocrionpathic laminitis and EMS. Early identification of diseased and at risk individuals is essential due to the limited therapeutic options for causal therapy, and the assessment of already slightly impaired insulin regulation is the crux of the matter. Oral glycemic challenges are currently recommended for assessing ID and, thereby, identifying pathological postprandial hyperinsulinemia under standardized conditions (Bertin and De Laat 2017; Durham et al. 2019).

The results of this research project indicate the importance of the exact quantification of equine insulin. The first part of this research project highlights the importance of the careful selection of the immunoassay used for the analyses of equine insulin and highlights the strengths and weaknesses of three commonly used and investigated assays. Although the measurement of equine insulin is one of the last steps in the clinical approach to diagnose ID or IR, it remains the most challenging part. Based on the study conducted in part II of this research project, it was possible to provide a clinically useful diagnostic approach to assess ID in combination with a reliable immunoassay-based quantification of equine insulin. However, insulin analysis with the equine-optimized porcine-specific ELISA (Equine Insulin ELISA, Mercodia AB) is not widely available in commercial laboratories and has the decisive disadvantage that it can not easily be performed on automated systems allowing high day-to-day variable sample volume.

Furthermore, testing for ID with oral test protocols focuses primarily on the assessment of standardized postprandial hyperinsulinemia and not direct on assessment of tissue IR. Therefore, dynamic IV testing protocols may provide a case-dependent advantage by assessing the insulin-mediated glucose uptake in insulin-dependent target tissues triggered by an injection of exogenous insulin and glucose as a substrate allowing the diagnosis off tissue IR. The study performed in part III of this research project evaluated assay-specific variations in the insulin concentrations supplied considering testing for ID with OGT or IR based on CGIT. Again, marked assay-specific differences in the insulin concentrations supplied occurred between the equine-optimized porcine-specific ELISA (Equine Insulin ELISA, Mercodia AB) already investigated previously and a human-specific IRMA (Insulin(e) IRMA KIT, Beckman Coulter). These findings preclude the interchangeable use of both and, together with the results from the study in part I, highlight the consideration of the immunoassay used for quantification in terms of the interpretation of laboratory findings in basal or resting samples as well as after stimulation with dynamic testing for PO and IV testing protocols.

Diagnosing ID by analyses of basal or resting samples collected from horses or ponies is the simplest diagnostic approach. The feeding regime prior to testing is currently discussed controversially in the group of experts in equine endocrinology (Bertin et al. 2016, Knowles et al. 2017, Durham et al. 2019). However, this research project indicates that, in addition to optimal and standardized pretesting conditions, the selection of the immunoassay method is as equally important as the pretesting conditions. Differences between insulin concentrations in basal blood samples measured with the various assays used in the current research project in part I and part III indicated striking and highly significant differences. Even the consideration of laboratory-specific reference ranges did not allow the identical classification as "healthy" or "insulin-dysregulated" in all cases. Insulin concentrations, for example, differed by a factor of 6.5 between the human-specific CLIA investigated (ADVIA Centaur XP, Siemens Healthcare Diagnostics) and equine-optimized porcine-specific ELISA (Equine Insulin ELISA, Mercodia AB), and a factor of 6 between the CLIA and the porcine-specific RIA (Porcine Insulin RIA, Merck Millipore) in one case.

Based on the simplicity, several studies evaluated and established cutoff values and reference ranges for basal or resting insulin. The reference for basal insulin concentrations most cited and clinically widely used is above 20 μIU/mL (Frank et al. 2010, Equine Endocrinology Group 2018). However, the cutoff was initially established in a cohort of ponies, which had been off pasture for one to three hours, by using a human-specific RIA (Coat-a-Count RIA, Diagnostic Products Corporation, Los Angeles, California, USA) (Treiber et al. 2006; Carter et al. 2009). As this assay is no longer available, the reference ranges had to be redefined on other immunoassays. Thus, the Equine Endocrinology Group (2018) classified insulin concentrations below 20 μIU/mL measured on a human-specific CLIA (IMMULITE 1000, Siemens Healthcare Diagnostics) as non-diagnostic, concentrations between 20 and 50 μIU/mL as suspicious, and concentrations above 50 μIU/mL as indicative of ID. However, they pointed out that the corresponding ranges differ when samples were analyzed by another human-specific CLIA (IMMULITE 2000xpi, Siemens Healthcare Diagnostics) and the respective values were 31 and 80 μIU/mL instead of 20 and 50 μIU/mL. Interestingly, **Koeller et al.** (2016) sampled 112 ponies with free access to hay and calculated a reference interval of 2.0–21.1 μIU/mL based on analyses with another human-specific CLIA (IMMULITE 2000, Siemens Healthcare Diagnostics) belonging to the same assay family. Thus, there is even evidence for a difference between the three IMMULITE[®] CLIAs. Furthermore, the similar range of insulin concentrations suggested around 20 μIU/mL used as a cutoff value for basal insulin by analyses with the human-specific RIA (Coat-a-Count RIA, Diagnostic Products Corporation) (Treiber et al. 2006; Carter et al. 2009) and the human-specific CLIA (IMMULITE 2000, Siemens Healthcare Diagnostics) is questionable based on the results of Carslake et al. (2017). This study investigated both immunoassays and reported that the CLIA tends to provide marked lower insulin concentrations in the analytical range of the cutoff values reported compared to the human-specific RIA. Considering the striking differences observed in part I and III of this research project in combination with the current data from literature, it can be concluded that there is a need to interpret the basal insulin concentrations carefully regarding the immunoassay used for quantification. Furthermore, there is evidence of uncertainty in using some of the basal cutoff values and reference ranges established previously.

Despite the large number of different immunoassays which have been investigated in the past, most veterinary laboratories currently use human-specific CLIA systems. The analyses of insulin with immunoassays can generally be complex, time-consuming and costly depending on the assay used. However, analyses on automated systems provide the substantial benefit that subsequent steps are performed automatically by the system and, therefore, reduce the risk of operator errors during different steps of the assay implementation. In these automated systems, samples were dispensed, followed by automated selection and dispensation of the reagent, incubation, separation from bound and free agents, dispensation of the substrate and, finally, reading of the signal provoked (Babson 2013, Metzar 2013). Currently, CLIAs are widely available for automated systems and human diagnostics. By contrast, only a few specific CLIAs designed for veterinary purposes are available. Most of these were designed for important infectious diseases of companion and food animals. Only a limited number of non-human species-specific CLIAs are commercially available for tests of metabolic functions, such as canine thyroid hormones (Iversen et al. 1999; Marca et al. 2001; Piechotta et al. 2010). Interestingly, no assay is available for any equine disease. Thus, immunoassays originally designed for human diagnostic purposes are used frequently in veterinary medicine despite the fact, that potential assay interference may occur or underlying assay antibodies are not compatible with epitopes of the animal species-specific conformation of the analyte.

Systems widely used for determination of equine insulin in veterinary medicine are based on the IMMULITE® family: IMMULITE 1000, IMMULITE 2000 and IMMULITE 2000xpi (Babson 2013). Despite belonging to the same system family, marked differences in the insulin concentrations supplied have occurred, as has already been mentioned (Banse et al. 2014, Koeller et al. 2016, Carslake et al. 2017, Durham et al. 2019). Moreover, these differences were not only limited to samples with relatively low insulin concentrations occurring in basal or resting samples. Furthermore, cutoff values for the oral sugar test (OST), a simplified oral glycemic challenge test, differ significantly, with a cutoff value of 40 µIU/mL calculated on analyses with the IMMULITE 1000 (Siemens Healthcare Diagnostics) and 63 µIU/mL using the IMMULITE 2000xpi (Siemens Healthcare Diagnostics) in a cohort of 35 ponies without a history of laminitis (Durham et al. 2019). The ADVIA Centaur XP system (Siemens Healthcare Diagnostics), another automated immunoassay system based on chemiluminescent, was used in part I of this research project. This system is widely used in commercial veterinary laboratories offering the measurement of insulin in equine samples. Despite frequent use, to the best of the author's knowledge, no further studies are available investigating the performance of this assay in equine serum samples. The comparison of this assay with a commonly used porcine-specific RIA (Porcine Insulin RIA, Millipore Merck) and the equine-optimized porcine-specific ELISA (Equine Insulin ELISA, Mercodia AB) performed in this research project showed significantly lower insulin concentrations in basal samples. In samples obtained during dynamic stimulation with PO glucose application with significantly higher insulin concentrations, the concentrations supplied still differed between the equine-optimized porcine-specific ELISA and the human-specific CLIA (ADVIA Centaur XP, Siemens Healthcare Diagnostics). However, the difference in insulin concentrations between the porcine-specific RIA and the human-specific CLIA did not reach significance. The human-specific CLIA provided lower results than the porcine-specific RIA for samples with concentrations under 100 µIU/mL but supplied higher results for five samples when the concentration exceeded 100 µIU/mL. This is in accordance with Carslake et al. (2017), who reported higher insulin concentrations supplied by another human-specific CLIA (IMMULITE 2000, Siemens Healthcare Diagnostics) compared to a human specific RIA (Coat-A-Count Insulin, Siemens Healthcare Diagnostics) in very high insulin ranges, in contrast to the opposite relationship in lower concentrations. These dynamic changes of bias between both assays might preclude simple comparison of insulin concentrations between the methods. From a clinician's point of view, this finding is even more important because insulin concentrations around 100 µIU/mL often occur in the diagnostic range for some dynamic stimulation tests. Jocelyn et al. (2018), for example, suggested an insulin concentration of above 110 µIU/mL measured by another human-specific RIA (Insulin CT, MP Biomedical) at 60 min post OST as a cutoff value for the identification of ID. In that respect, the cutoff value of 110 µIU/mL for the OGT procedure established in part II of this research project is in the same concentration range. Although, it has to be taken into consideration that the quantification of insulin was based on the equine-optimized porcine-specific ELISA in this research project.

Despite frequent use, reliable reference ranges for the OGT procedure performed via NGT have not yet been available. Therefore, the aim of the second part of this research project was to calculate a cutoff value for the standard dose OGT performed with NGT and subsequent insulin quantification with an appropriate immunoassay for the quantification of equine insulin. The generation of reference ranges or a cutoff value for a new diagnostic test or analytical method can be challenging and often requires great effort when performed correctly (Geffre et al. 2009). Per definition, a reference value is used to describe the dispersion of a variable in healthy individuals. Reference values are usually reported as population-based reference intervals comprising 95 % of the healthy population (Marshall and Bangert 2008). Taking into account international recommendations, the preferred method is an *a priori* nonparametric determination from at least 120 reference individuals, thus, requiring relatively large datasets with extensive documentation (Clinical and Laboratory Standards Institute 2008). This can be even more challenging in veterinary medicine (Geffre et al. 2009). In the case of the replacement of a diagnostic test by a new method, the new diagnostic test has to be compared to a gold standard test. Furthermore, transference of a reference interval requires a well-defined previous one, a comparable analytical system and comparable patient populations (Geffre et al. 2009). Though, two major limitations existed in this context. Firstly, there was no gold standard available to compare against the laboratory method used for the quantification of the equine insulin. Analyte detection and quantification based on HPLC-MS technology is often considered to be the most reliable technique and gold standard even in detection of steroid and peptide hormones (Stanczyk et al. 2010, Thevis et al. 2011). This technique enables detection based on physicochemical properties of the peptide and not on epitope

78

recognition (Anderson et al. 2006). Analysis of equine serum or plasma samples with the HPLC-MS method for quantification of equine insulin was performed by Tinworth et al. (2011). However, samples were previously prepared for HPLC-MS analysis using a protocol for the analysis of insulin in human urine (Thomas et al. 2009). In the latter protocol, anti-insulin antibodies are used for the initial capture of the insulin molecules and further processing of antigen-antibody aggregates. Therefore, results can be influenced by interference of the target analyte and antibody-specific capture epitope. In our experiments, the HPLC-MS technique was not available and comparison of the results supplied by the three immunoassays investigated in part I and part III against a more specific method, such as HPLC-MS, was not performed. Moreover, equine insulin standards used previously to evaluate the recovery of equine insulin in spiked samples, as was performed by Banse et al. (2014) and Carslake et al. (2017), was unavailable at the time the study was performed. However, based on the findings in part I with critically reevaluation of the equine-optimized porcine-specific insulin ELISA (Equine Insulin ELISA, Mercodia AB), indication of acceptable performance measures and satisfying clinically relevant differentiation of individuals, the following investigations and calculations regarding the definition of a reliable reference range for OGT have been based on insulin analyses with the equine-optimized porcine-specific ELISA. Moreover, the ELISAs satisfying performance data from part I were in line with further convincing data from other studies (Öberg et al. 2011, Borer-Weir et al. 2012).

Secondly, the results presented in part II of the research project support the hypothesis that insulin sensitivity is a dynamic condition and not a dichotomic state of being either insulin-sensitive or -dysregulated. It also supports the idea that impaired insulin regulation exists in different intensities. In fact, the insulin response to glucose is probably a continuum among all horses and ponies, whether or not they are described as healthy or dysregulated. This finding, together with the lack of a gold standard to compare against, complicated the definition of a reference range or cutoff value.

Therefore, a model-based clustering method was used to circumvent the use of an arbitrary limit for categorization. This method considered all data-points for the classification, taking into account the individual insulin trajectory during the OGT. A strength of the analyses and the study is that repeated blood samples over a period of three hours have been included in the clustering method. In total, insulin concentrations during the course of 13 samples per animal have been considered for cluster analysis. Two clusters were differentiated with this method, one with low and one with high insulin responses during OGT. The cluster of individuals with low insulin response was consistently detected, independently of the initialization parameters of the algorithm. Based on the low cluster, the 97.5 % quantile of insulin was 110 µLU/mL at 120 min and then used as a cutoff value. With data from 56 horses and ponies undergoing OGT, the cutoff generated in the part II of this research project is based on a larger sample set than previously published and suggested cutoffs for dynamic testing for ID. Nevertheless, the suggested cutoff value is only valid in the case of considering the combination of the specific dynamic test protocol for the OGT via NGT in combination with the corresponding insulin quantification with the equine-optimized porcine-specific insulin ELISA (Equine Insulin ELISA, Mercodia AB). Comparison across immunoassays will still remain challenging based on the marked differences between the insulin concentrations supplied by the different assays reported in part I and III.

Another finding in part II of this research project is the wide dynamic ranges of insulinemic responses after the application of glucose via NGT. These variations between individuals may also provide additional diagnostic information. Horses showed monophasic and biphasic insulin secretion patterns, which is in accordance with previous studies reporting both after oral glucose challenge (Schuver et al. 2014; Smith et al. 2016). However, a potential difference in the secretion pattern of insulin between insulin-sensitive and insulin-dysregulated animals is often the subject of debate. Despite the fact that frequent re-sampling of the animal tested to increase the diagnostic accuracy of the test may not be practically feasible in a clinical situation, differences in the secretion pattern might influence the optimal time point for the collection of the most reliable diagnostic sample. Whereas insulin-sensitive individuals responded with fast increases in the insulin concentrations and early peak concentrations, insulin-dysregulated individuals responded with a more continuously increase and later achievement of peak concentrations. The optimal time point for sample collection may remain a subject of further research, but so far, the time point of 120 min previously defined and used allowed a satisfactory differentiation in the present study population. The difference between the determined clusters in part II even increased with time after glucose application and later sampling time points. Whereas severely dysregulated animals still increased in insulin concentrations after 120 to 180 min, the insulin-sensitive animals had already returned to basal insulin concentrations. These findings reflect the effective regulation of glycemic control in insulin-sensitive individuals compared to the obviously dysregulated individuals with a significant imbalance between blood glucose concentration and β-cell-mediated insulinemic response. Hence, later sampling time points provide further diagnostic safety for differentiation between the insulin-sensitive and severe insulin-dysregulated individuals but may lack reliable identification of mild subclinical changes in animals being at risk of developing ID. Moreover, later sampling time points might be a disadvantage due to the time-consuming procedure for sample collection under clinical field conditions. Nevertheless, extended statistics and mathematical operations have been performed with data generated in part II of this research project to offer dynamic reference ranges during the OGT procedure with sample collection at variable time points between 90 and 180 min to further optimize and simplify the diagnostic procedure and assessment of ID under clinical conditions. Based on the current dataset, the extension of the period for sample collection defined previously was possible. The 97.5 % CI calculated based on the median insulin concentration observed in cluster one is not limited to a specific time point. Thus, the extension of the sample collection time period in a dynamic range was possible and, thereby, simplified the implementation of OGT under clinical settings by providing a more flexible blood sample collection time frame (www.ogt-reference-provider.org).

The early identification of animals at high risk of developing impaired insulin regulation towards ID must be a primary goal of the diagnostic approach. If hyperinsulinemia induced laminitis, changes developed in the lamellar-distal phalangeal attachment apparatus are irreversible (De Laat et al. 2010, De Laat et al.

2013, Patterson-Kane et al. 2018, De Laat 2019). So far, no convincing medical treatment options for ID have become available but recent research highlights the promising effects of sodium-glucose linked transport-2 inhibitors, such as velagliflozin (Meier et al. 2018; Meier et al. 2019). These potential new therapeutic options will encourage a debate on the thresholds and limits for advisement of drug-based treatment in contrast to sole management changes. In the future, the combination of clinical signs and evaluation of case outcome with the absolute insulin concentration during OGT might be considered as an indicator of a prognostic factor. De Laat et al. (2019) have already reported an association of higher basal insulin concentrations with more severe lameness in cases with endocrinopathic laminitis. In this context, Meier et al. (2017) performed a study to evaluate the important predictive significance mentioned previously of in-feed OGT testing for the identification of individual animals at high risk of developing laminitis based on their hyperinsulinemia. A predictive cutoff value of 65 µIU/mL generated by in-feed OGT performed with 1 g/kg BW was reported for the differentiation of ponies becoming laminitic or not under an experimentally performed laminitis induction model based on a high NSC diet challenge. The serum samples in this study have been analyzed with the human-specific CLIA (ADVIA Centaur XP, Siemens Healthcare Diagnostics) also being investigated in part I of this research project. Keeping in mind the marked lower insulin concentrations supplied by this assay compared to the equine-optimized porcine-specific ELISA (Equine Insulin ELISA, Mercodia AB), the study shows strong accordance with the results reported in part II of this research project. When comparing the calculated cutoff value of 110 µIU/mL established in insulin analyses with the equine-optimized porcine-specific ELISA by use of the equation from regression analysis ($Y = 0.3909^* \times +0.4002$) to the human-specific CLIA (ADVIA Centaur XP, Siemens Healthcare Diagnostics) data, the transferred cutoff value for the CLIA corresponds to 43 µIU/mL. Taking this as a basis, the cutoff value generated from part II of the study still implies a safety zone. Taking it the other way around, the suggested predictive cutoff value of 65 µIU/mL established in the CLIA (ADVIA Centaur XP, Siemens Healthcare Diagnostics) corresponds to around 160 µIU/mL in the equine-optimized porcine-specific ELISA. Thus, the prediction of the incidence of laminitis in the clinical study with the diet model fits to the cutoff value established in part II of the study. Furthermore, a combination of conclusions of both studies allow further prognostic classification of ID cases tested with the OGT via NGT as being at high risk for the development of laminitis in cases of insulin concentrations above 160 µIU/mL.

The calculated cutoff value in part II of the study is based on retrospective analyses of insulin responses during OGT procedures of various horse and pony breeds and, therefore, represents a species wide, general orientation value. Backtracking to primary literature of several suggested cutoff values for ID or IR reported in review articles for a closer inspection of underlying data with respect to the breed composition of the study population was impossible in most cases (Frank 2011; Frank and Geor 2014; Bertin and De Laat 2017; Durham et al. 2019). Although it is widely acknowledged that ID is common in certain breeds and rare in other breeds (Frank et al. 2010, Durham et al. 2019), this project used a mixed cohort of animals. Some studies reported significant breed differences in insulin regulation (Bamford et al. 2014, Duehlmeier et al. 2001) with different glucose and insulin kinetics (Smith et al. 2016, Cantarelli et al. 2018). In the same line, Manfredi (2016) identified differences in the optimal cutoff and sampling time point for the OST procedure in Arabians, Morgans, Welsh Ponies, Quarter Horses and Thoroughbreds. However, subgroups of individuals used for the calculation of thresholds for ID and optimal time point for sample collection ranged from six to twenty-two individuals in that study. By contrast, Lindase et al. (2016) did not detect differences in the OST between Shetland ponies, Icelandic horses and Thoroughbreds. Thus, there is currently no consensus regarding the breed-related impact. Subdividing the mixed population used in part II of the study to calculate breed-specific reference ranges for OGT was impossible due to the number of remaining animals per group being too low. Nevertheless, the distribution of breeds was equal between the clusters without overrepresentation of a certain breed in one cluster. Thus, the study population represents a representative cross section of patients being presented to a veterinarian for evaluation of ID.

In general, the number of animals and their selection or classification as ID or IS used for calculating reference ranges or cutoff values remains the most limiting factor when reviewing the literature critically. A larger number of animals are favored to calculate reliable reference ranges or cutoff values (Geffre et al. 2009), but most of the time, the number of animals are very low. In addition, their classification criteria *per se* or the classification criteria as healthy or diseased may be reviewed critically in some publications.

Commonly, OGTs with NGT have been performed in clinical settings without the awareness that reliable reference ranges are lacking. Often cutoff values or reference ranges generated for in-feed OGT or OST have been used for the interpretation of insulin concentrations from OGT via NGT without considering the specific differences in testing protocols due to missing data. However, there are simple but physiological important differences between the tests. Smith et al. (2016) reported differences in glucose and insulin kinetics when comparing OST and in-feed OGT and explained the differences observed between OST and in-feed OGT by the differences in administration techniques. Whereas the corn syrup was given as an oral bolus, the glucose powder was mixed in chaff and offered for voluntary uptake by trough feeding. Thus, this explanation is in line with Mair et al. (1991), who identified meal size and starch content as factors altering the rate of gastric emptying, with higher starch and larger meals emptying most slowly. In OGT via NGT, the glucose is bypassed by the oral cavity, solved in water and, therefore, might have increased gastric passage based on simple physiological features. These basic differences may already provide less stimulation compared to the voluntary uptake of a meal artificially enriched with glucose by which the process of ingestion provides the stimulation of sweet taste receptors in the oral cavity and may produce an already triggered state when glucose is entering the small intestine (De Graaf-Roelfsema 2014, De Laat et al. 2016a).

There are multiple arguments for and against specific test protocols for the implementation of oral dynamic testing for ID. The potential stress influence of NGT insertion during the OGT procedure, for example, is a common concern. Cortisol increased after glucose application via NGT during the OGT procedure in healthy horses but returned back to baseline levels after 90 min (Warnken et al. 2018), therefore, questioning the impact of hypothalamic-hypophysic-adrenal (HPA) axis activation. In another study investigating the activation of HPA axis during OGT and sham OGT in healthy and insulin dysregulated ponies, a significant increase in ACTH and cortisol directly after insertion and removal of the NGT in the OGT and sham OGT procedure was observed but did not result in any clinically relevant variation in insulin and glucose concentrations in the sham OGT procedure (Warnken et al. 2017). Nevertheless, the direct influence on OGT-related glucose kinetics by activation of the HPA axis remains unknown. Incomplete ingestion is the most important issue complicating the diagnostic procedure during in-feed OGTs. De Laat and Sillence (2017) reported partial refused feed intake of up to 70 % in 5 out of 12 ponies when using standard dose 1 g/kg BW glucose for in-feed OGT. Clinical experience is in accordance with these reports, often limiting clinical usability of the in-feed OGT and requiring reappointment and implementation of an alternative diagnostic test, such as the OGT with glucose application via NGT. Therefore, the focus of this research project was on the OGT via NGT providing a reliable, exact and quick administration of a specific amount of glucose avoiding potential impact by other factors like for example prolonged ingestion time.

Despite many advantages, recent experiments indicated that application of 1 g/kg BW glucose for the implementation of OGT might not be the ideal dosage. Kenez et al. (2018) reported a pro-inflammatory shift reflected by increased kynurenine and decreased spermidine concentrations during the OGT procedure because of hyperstimulation of the metabolic system. This highlights the question concerning the optimal amount of glycemic stimulus needed for reliable diagnostics. It has been shown for in-feed OGT that 0.75 g/kg BW glucose supplied sufficient glycemic and insulinemic responses to differentiate between insulin-dysregulated and healthy equids (De Laat and Sillence 2017). Furthermore, the postprandial insulinemic responses after in-feed OGT performed with 0.75 g/kg BW glucose and 2 h post-grazing was positively correlated, thus, proving evidence to support the suitability of standardized oral glycemic challenge tests as clinically significant test models (Fitzgerald et al. 2019b). In accordance with this finding, debates regarding the ideal dosages for OST are the subject of current discussions. Initially, Schuver et al. (2014) suggested 0.15 ml/kg BW corn syrup as an appropriate dosage. By contrast, the opposing discussion to the OGT-related one aiming for a reduction of the comparatively high glucose amount aiming for an increase in glycemic stimulation takes place for OST. Recent studies investigated the optimal glycemic stimulation for the implementation of OST and suggested higher glycemic stimulation, achieved by increased amounts of 0.25 or 0.45 ml/kg BW corn syrup to increase sensitivity and specificity of the test (Manfredi 2016; Jacob et al. 2018a; Jocelyn et al. 2018). This dosage discussion is highly important considering the marked difference between the various immunoassays used for the measurement of the equine insulin in samples obtained during these testing procedures. By lowering the glycemic stimulation and, therefore, reducing the glycemic and insulinemic responses in healthy and diseased animals, the immunoassay performance is essential for a reliable detection of diseased individuals and may be a limiting factor. By lowering the insulinemic response, the expected concentration range in samples obtained during the testing procedure is shifted towards the lower parts of the analytical range and calibration curve. Exactly this may necessitate satisfying quantification and differentiation in relatively low insulin concentration ranges to still detect differences between healthy insulin-sensitive individuals and insulin-dysregulated ones. Therefore, the analytical range of the assay, the LLOD and the performance in the lower assay range is crucial. The results from part I of this research project clearly indicate that the three investigated immunoassays have variable performance at the lower area of the analytical range. Especially immunoassays such as the human-specific CLIA (ADVIA Centaur XP, Siemens Healthcare Diagnostics) which reported constantly lower insulin concentrations compared to more widespread and differentiated concentrations reported by other assays might reach their limits.

Commonly, intra- and inter-assay CVs increase with decreased analyte concentrations at the lower analytical range of the assay (Davies 2013), thereby, procuring more improper results. Considering the high CVs for low insulin concentrations reported for several immunoassays, the trend towards the suggestion of lower cutoffs might be even more challenging. Thus, it is important to take into account that combinations of testing protocols and immunoassay methods used for analyses of samples obtained during dynamic testing can increase or decrease test sensitivity. Identifying concentrations at one end of the analytical range of the assay is always challenging and a cause of variation, whereas measurement of analyte concentrations ranging in the mean analytical range are most reliable.

This is not only a problem during dynamic testing but also in analyses of basal samples. Based on the comparison of basal, fasted insulin concentrations to CGIT results, Olley et al. (2019) suggested a downward adjustment of the initial fasted insulin cutoff of 20 µIU/mL towards a more sensitive cutoff of 5.2 µIU/mL based on analyses of insulin with the human-specific CLIA IMMULITE 2000 (IMMULITE 2000, Siemens Healthcare Diagnostics). This might be possible due to the excellent precision of IMMULITE 2000 for low insulin concentrations reported by Carslake et al. (2017) but might be more difficult or not possible with immunoassays having higher CVs for low equine insulin concentrations, such as IMMULITE 1000 (IMMULITE 1000, Siemens Healthcare Diagnostics) (Banse et al. 2014) or other assays. Nevertheless, reliable differentiation between insulin sensitive and insulin dysregulated individuals requires clear distinction that might not be achieved in all cases with assays reporting generally very low insulin concentrations. In part I of this research project the ELISA (Equine Insulin ELISA, Mercodia AB) and the RIA (Porcine Insulin RIA, Millipore Merck) were able to differentiate the measured basal, fasted samples in a range from 2.4 µIU/mL to 72.7 µIU/mL (median: 13.3 µIU/mL) and 3.4 µIU/mL to 57.0 µIU/mL (median: 19.3 µIU/mL), respectively, whereas the CLIA (ADVIA Centaur XP, Siemens Healthcare Diagnostics) failed to accurately discriminate the variable insulin concentrations over a broad range by reporting insulin concentrations ranging from 1.0 µIU/mL to 32.2 µIU/mL (median:5.34 µIU/mL). Thus, the diagnostic accuracy might be lowered or limited in cases were immunoassays with a narrow level of differentiation were used for quantification of insulin.

Summarizing the testing for ID still remains a subject of ongoing research to identify the optimal and most reliable protocol regarding clinical applicability. In the future, further harmonization of testing protocols would be as important as the harmonization of the measurement of insulin. Harmonization of laboratory-based measurements of insulin would indicate that comparable results would be obtained independent of when and where the analysis is performed. In human medicine, several studies have been performed to investigate difference between methods and to standardize methods for quantification of human insulin (Marcovina et al. 2007, Miller et al. 2009, Staten et al. 2010). Based on the high number of variable protocols, it is not realistic that all commercial veterinary laboratories offer laboratory- and immunoassay-specific reference ranges for all tests. Further research is needed either to allow the transformation of previously defined cutoff values to other methods or to generate cutoff values or reference ranges for specific test protocols with variable immunoassay methods to enable global operation. Given the fact that specialists in equine endocrinology cannot reach an agreement on a standardized recommended diagnostic approach and a reference laboratory method, it is our duty to provide substantial information to enable diagnoses of ID.

According to general recommendations, comparison between immunoassay methods should be based on high sample numbers and broad ranges of clinically significant analyte concentrations (American Society for Veterinary Clinical Pathology 2009). This is not always achieved when reviewing the relevant literature or critically considering part I of this research project with a limited number of 40 samples used for comparison. In part III of this research project, a more satisfying number of 268 serum samples has been used for comparison. In addition to the simple comparison between the equine-optimized procine-specific ELISA (Equine Insulin ELISA, Mercodia AB) and the human-specific IRMA (Insulin(e) IRMA KIT, Beckman Coulter), the data were analyzed with a special focus on the presence of endogenous equine insulin present after PO glucose application in OGT and the presence of exogenous non-equine insulin after IV injection in the GCIT procedure. Again, the equine-optimized porcine-specific ELISA (Equine Insulin ELISA, Mercodia AB) showed satisfying assay performance similar to the human-specific IRMA (Insulin(e) IRMA KIT, Beckman Coulter), with acceptable CVs, good linearity of dilution and recovery upon dilution.

Both assays supplied significantly different insulin concentrations for the same sample in samples obtained during the OGT procedure. The human-specific IRMA (Insulin(e) IRMA KIT, Beckman Coulter) gave constantly higher concentrations compared to the equine-optimized porcine-specific ELISA (Equine Insulin ELISA, Mercodia AB), with a proportional increase with increased average insulin concentration. Despite the fact that the assays supplied markedly different insulin concentrations, regression analyses indicated a strong linear relationship. However, the proportional error between both methods again precluded simple conversion with multiplication of results by a certain factor. The fact that the human-specific IRMA supplied markedly higher insulin concentrations in basal samples and samples obtained during the dynamic stimulation might be critical for the interpretation with currently established cutoff values. Transformation of the cutoff value calculated for OGT via NGT in part II to the human-specific IRMA (Insulin(e) IRMA KIT, Beckman Coulter) by use of the regression analysis (Y = 2.081* x -1.751) resulted in an adapted cutoff value of 227 µIU/mL. This major difference in the absolute insulin value of 110 µIU/mL in the equine-optimized ELISA (Equine Insulin ELISA, Mercodia AB) and 227 µIU/mL in the human-specific IRMA (Insulin(e) IRMA KIT, Beckman Coulter) highlights the importance of assay consideration when interpreting the laboratory data for diagnosing ID in the OGT procedure via NGT. Based on the current investigations performed with both assays, it is not possible to state whether the equine-optimized porcine-specific ELISA (Equine Insulin ELISA, Mercodia AB) or the human-specific IRMA (Insulin(e) IRMA KIT, Beckman Coulter) detects equine insulin more reliably. As mentioned earlier the human-specific IRMA might be applicable and advantageous if the glycemic stimuli in a certain PO test protocol is very low or should be reduced and, therefore, small changes in the individual's insulinemic response have to be detected.

Similar to the case regarding diagnosing ID, several testing protocols have been established for the detection of IR (Garcia and Beech 1986, Hoffman et al. 2003, Eiler et al. 2005, Pratt et al. 2005, Treiber et al. 2005, Caltabilota et al. 2010, Bertin and Sojka-Kritchevsky 2013) but the HEC remains the gold standard for the assessment of tissue IR (Rijnen and Van Der Kolk 2003, Kronfeld et al. 2005, Pratt et al. 2005, Pratt-Phillips et al. 2015). This test may not be practical under clinical conditions due to the complexity of implementation and is, therefore, mainly reserved for research purposes. However, simplified procedures have been established. Out of all the protocols for the detection of IR, the CGIT remains the most suitable test for a practical approach when considering and balancing the effort and the diagnostic value. Therefore, the CGIT was used in part III of this research project as a model to provide equine serum samples mainly containing exogenous non-equine insulin. In accordance with the samples obtained during the OGT procedure, the insulin concentrations measured with the equine-optimized porcine-specific ELISA (Equine Insulin ELISA, Mercodia AB) and the human-specific RIA (Insulin(e) IRMA KIT, Beckman Coulter) differed significantly in these CGIT samples. Most laboratories process serum samples obtained during CGIT in a similar way to samples obtained during PO tests. However, the analyte of interest, endogenous equine insulin or exogenous non-equine insulin might be different. The diagnosis of IR during CGIT is based mainly on the assessment of the insulin-mediated glucose kinetics (Eiler et al. 2005; Frank et al. 2010; Durham et al. 2019). Nevertheless, additional diagnostic information is based on the clearance of insulin from plasma within 45 min. Eiler et al. (2005) considered insulin concentrations after 45 min less than 100 µIU/mL as being indicative of IR. Due to the simultaneous application of glucose and high amounts of exogenous insulin, it could be assumed that the endogenous insulin secretion is initially suppressed. Therefore, samples collected in the early period of the CGIT contain mainly exogenous insulin and only small amounts of endogenous equine insulin. In these samples, potential cross-reactivity due to the presence of endogenous equine insulin and exogenously injected non-equine insulin or insulin analogues complicate the analyses. Eiler et al. (2005) established the CGIT test protocol with use of a recombinant human insulin. Subsequent sample analysis in the original publication was then performed with a human-specific RIA (Coat-A-Count, Diagnostic Products Corp). Therefore, 100 % of the injected human insulin should have been detected during analyses. To date, various insulin formulations and analogues have been licensed in veterinary medicine for the treatment of diabetes in cats and dogs (e.g. protamine zinc-insulin as ProZinc® 40 IU/mL Boehringer

Ingelheim Vetmedica GmbH, Ingelheim, Germany, or porcine zinc-insulin as Caninsulin® 40 IU/mL, MSD, Unterschleißheim, Germany). Therefore, CGITs were sometimes performed with these analogues instead of regular recombinant human insulin. Insulin analogues are characterized by substitutions at various amino acids or additions of residues to the COOH terminus of the B-chain for impairment of their pharmacokinetics for special issues like e.g. short- or long-acting properties. These modifications, however, can also alter antigen-antibody binding in immunoassays if present at the antibodies specific binding epitope. In the third part of this research project, porcine zinc-insulin was used for the implementation of the CGIT thus providing samples with high amounts of exogenous non-equine insulin for comparison of two immunoassay methods. Based on the fact that the equine-optimized porcine-specific ELISA (Equine Insulin ELISA, Mercodia AB) is based on antibodies directed against epitopes of the porcine insulin molecule, it was suspected of detect 100 % of the injected exogenous porcine insulin with this assay and therefore resulting in higher insulin concentrations measured with this assay compared to the human-specific IRMA (Insulin(e) IRMA KIT, Beckman Coulter). In contrast to the expectation, the human-specific IRMA (Insulin(e) IRMA KIT, Beckman Coulter) supplied even higher insulin concentrations compared to the ELISA. No information about the specific target epitope of the antibodies used in ELISA and IRMA is publicly accessible. In conclusion, the underlying mechanism provoking the higher concentrations in the human-specific IRMA (Insulin(e) IRMA KIT, Beckman Coulter) could not be explained based on the current data of this research project and needs further investigation. In line with this, further investigation is needed to evaluate the impact of the presence of exogenous non-equine insulin in samples from CGITs when being analyzed with various immunoassay methods to critically evaluate the additional sense of purpose of the determination of insulin at 45 min during CGIT. Currently, descriptive data for insulin and glucose kinetics during CGIT is only available for porcine zinc-insulin measured with the ELISA (Equine Insulin ELISA, Mercodia AB) which has been investigated in the present research project (Warnken et al. 2018) but not for human protamine zinc-insulin. Moreover, there is no further data available comparing the potential interference of the injected insulin formulation during CGIT with the immunoassay used for sample analyzes, despite the results presented in part III of this research project. In contrast to the situation in equine medicine, studies in human medicine investigated the potential interference and reported marked impairment of insulin analyses by the presence of insulin analogues in patients treated for diabetes type 1 (Owen and Roberts 2004; Dayaldasani et al. 2015). High cross-reactivity was present when investigated for the IMMULITE® systems (IMMULITE, Siemens Healthcare Diagnostics) and the ADVIA Centaur XP systems (ADVIA Centaur XP, Siemens Healthcare Diagnostics); both assays being frequently used in veterinary medicine as well. Depending on the insulin analogue present and the immunoassay used, the cross-reactivity in human samples was reported ranging from 42 to 152 % (Owen and Roberts 2004). This, therefore, raises the question: What would be mainly measured in samples obtained from CGITs and analyzed with these assays. Further studies are needed to evaluate firstly the impact of insulin formulation used for CGIT and the corresponding pharmacokinetics and –dynamics and secondly the impact of these insulin formulations on the quantification by frequently used immunoassays. Until now, veterinarians should be aware that the insulin or insulin analogue used in CGIT might alter test results depending on the cross-reactivity in the immunoassay method used for analysis. When performed with human recombinant insulin, sample analyzes with a human specific immunoassay method might provide most reliable concentrations from a laboratory point of view. On the other hand, the clinical interpretation for diagnosis of IR remains challenging until CGIT reference ranges for other immunoassay methods than the one used in the original publication have been established.

Summing up, quantification of equine insulin in diagnostic procedure for assessment of ID and IR remains the most limiting step in the accuracy of the diagnosis and requires knowledge of immunoassay specific performance parameters for reliable interpretation.

9 CONCLUSION

Equine metabolic syndrome is a significant problem and health concern in the equine population and has severe welfare considerations. It can be assumed that the prevalence of EMS and the major laboratory key finding ID will increase in the future based on the development of the equine industry and population. Therefore, further investigations to reveal the underlying pathomechanisms behind ID and the common sequel endocrinopathic laminitis is urgently required. Diagnosing ID will remain challenging under clinical settings unless the further harmonization of diagnostic approaches and quantification is achieved. Based on the high number of variable diagnostic test protocols, it is not realistic that all commercial veterinary laboratories offer laboratory- and immunoassay-specific reference ranges for all tests. So far, quantification of equine insulin has remained a limiting step when evaluating different diagnostic tests for the assessment of ID or IR unless comparison of all available assays and information regarding their possible advantages and disadvantages in combination with specific diagnostic protocols is publicly accessible. This having been said, the present research project provides and summarizes a compilation of at least some of the different immunoassay comparisons with provision of data for conversion of insulin concentrations supplied by different immunoassays and for the transformation of previously defined reference ranges between immunoassay methods. However, diagnostic tests must be evaluated critically based on their physiological mode of action and limitations. This particularly highlights their clinical applicability. Finally, most cases were seen as first-opinion cases in fields, thus, requiring simple, efficient, quick, cost-effective and, most importantly, reliable diagnostic tests.

The main conclusion from this research project is that insulin concentrations measured by different immunoassays need to be interpreted carefully for making a clinical decision or diagnosis. Insulin concentrations obtained as results of basal or dynamic testing should be interpreted considering the immunoassay used whenever possible. Moreover, reevaluation of cases with serial sampling or testing for the control of therapeutic success or improved ID due to constructive and effective management changes should ideally be performed with the same immunoassay method to allow comparison. This will be particularly important if further medical treatment options become widely available. Apart from that, immunoassays with reported differences to immunoassays established previously should not automatically be blacklisted. Some may provide substantial benefits for specific diagnostic approaches but may lack specific features for others. Thus, a clever combination of immunoassays and diagnostic test protocols may provide a basis for the assessment of ID with mutual compensation of deficits taking full advantage of available options.

As veterinarians acting with responsibility, it is our obligation to provide substantial information to enable diagnoses of ID and prevent potential life-threatening laminitis in as many cases as possible.

10 FUTURE PERSPECTIVES

Quantification of equine insulin will remain challenging. From economical perspectives, development of immunoassays based on antibodies directed against specific epitopes of the equine insulin molecule is not attractive. However, this would solve many problems with assessment of ID and IR in equids. In the meantime, further comparison studies may provide substantial knowledge on the performance, advantages, disadvantages and main limitations of various immunoassays used for analyses of equine insulin. This allows further comparison of results from research studies to facilitate focused research progress without losing power and information based on the matter of fact that comparison of results is impossible due to massive differences in methodology. Being one-step ahead and taking a look into the ongoing research in human medicine, further investigation in combination of multiple parameters as a diagnostic panel might increase the test sensitivity and specificity and potentially simplifies the diagnostic approach. In line with this, the identification of potential biomarkers for ID might be another possible option to circumvent diagnostic testing and quantification of equine insulin with all its problems and limitations. Yet there are few studies performed in horses and ponies reporting interesting findings and specific markers for either EMS in general or specific assessment if ID by performance of metabolomics or sophisticated statistical approaches handling large datasets (Jacob et al. 2018b, Kenez et al. 2018, Lewis et al. 2018). Further investigation of these markers by the different research groups might also make dynamic testing redundant in the future and allow simple basal testing with high sensitivity and specificity. However, until then further research is needed to investigate the relation and potentially clinically significant association between high insulin responses during standardized PO glycemic challenges and clinical outcome of EMS cases. This may allow a more specific therapeutic approach and prognostic assessment in the future. Finally as already mentioned dynamic test protocols like PO glycemic challenge should be further optimized in regards of the optimal and needed quantity of the glycemic stimuli, the formulation of the glycemic challenger and the method of application or delivery.

11 SUMMARY

Tobias Warnken

Comparison of various methods for quantification of equine insulin under clinical settings for assessment of insulin dysregulation

Equine Metabolic Syndrome is an increasing problem and health concern in the equine population. Recent research suggests that ID with concurrent hyperinsulinemia is the only one among the cluster of signs and symptoms that characterize EMS that is clearly linked to the most common sequel, the development of endocrinopathic laminitis. Insulin dysregulation can manifest in several ways, including basal hyperinsulinemia, an excessive or prolonged hyperinsulinemic response to PO, or IV carbohydrate challenge and/or tissue IR.

The assessment of ID can be challenging, time-consuming and costly in clinical settings. However, it can be achieved by the use of basal or resting blood samples or multiple dynamic stimulation tests focusing on either the identification of ID or tissue IR. Oral glycemic challenges are currently recommended to assess ID and, thereby, identify postprandial hyperinsulinemia under standardized conditions. Most of the diagnostic procedures are based on the analysis of insulin concentrations in equine blood samples. However, previous studies indicated marked differences in insulin concentrations obtained from sample analyses with different commonly used immunoassays. It is important to mention that most immunoassays used in veterinary medicine were originally designed for human diagnostics and, thus, are based on antibodies directed against human insulin. Although there is a high sequence homology in vertebrates, the amino acid sequences between equine and human insulin differ.

Therefore, the main objective of this research project was, firstly, to evaluate the quantification of equine insulin considering the clinical demands and conditions and, secondly, to optimize the assessment of equine ID by a combination of appropriate dynamic diagnostic testing and quantification of equine insulin with a compatible and reliable immunoassay.

The aim of the first part of this research project was to compare three commonly used immunoassays for the analysis of equine insulin with a special focus on their assay performance and clinical applicability in assessing ID. This was achieved, firstly, by the analysis of basal blood samples and, secondly, by analyses of blood samples obtained during an OGT with glucose application via NCG which provoked elevated insulin concentrations resulting in a broad range of variable insulin concentrations in the samples. The assays investigated are an equine-optimized porcine-specific insulin ELISA, a porcine-specific insulin RIA and a human-specific insulin CLIA. All of them are frequently used for the measurement of equine insulin in commercial veterinary laboratories. Insulin concentrations obtained by the three investigated immunoassays from the analyses of basal blood samples differed significantly. Analyses of samples obtained during OGT with consecutively higher insulin concentrations revealed significantly lower insulin concentrations supplied by the human-specific CLIA compared to the equine-optimized porcine-specific ELISA. In conclusion, the results indicated that insulin concentrations measured in the same sample by different immunoassays vary greatly and should be interpreted carefully. Consideration of the immunoassay used for the quantification of the equine insulin and reliable assay-specific reference ranges or cut-off values are of particular importance and necessary for the clinical interpretation and diagnosing of ID. Based on these findings, the aim of the second part of this research project was formulated as further descriptions of variations in insulin responses to OGT via NGT and the calculation of a clinically useful cut-off value for the assessment of ID when quantifying the equine insulin with the previously validated equine-optimized insulin ELISA. Therefore, insulinemic responses of 56 horses and ponies after standard dosed OGT via NGT performed with the application of 1 g/kg BW glucose were analyzed retrospectively. Because initial data visualization revealed no clear separation of insulin-sensitive and insulin-dysregulated horses during the OGT, a model-based clustering method was used to circumvent the use of an arbitrary limit for categorization. This method accounted for the individual insulin trajectory during the OGT and differentiated two clusters, one with low and one with high insulin responses during OGT. The cluster of individuals with low insulin response was consistently detected, independently of the initialization parameters of the algorithm. Based on the 97.5 % quantile of insulin in this cluster, the cut-off value of 110 µIU/mL at 120 min was calculated. Thus, this research project provides the first cut-off value for the assessment of ID in horses based on the OGT procedure performed with 1 g/kg BW glucose and administration via NGT followed by the quantification of equine insulin by the equine-optimized porcine-specific ELISA.

Since the assessment of ID can also be based on the assessment of tissue IR, as one aspect of ID, a third research project was conducted and investigated the influence of insulin analyses performed with two immunoassays in samples obtained during the OGT procedure for the assessment of ID and in samples obtained during CGIT for the assessment of tissue IR. Despite the different underlying test mechanisms and physiological features, the quantification of equine insulin is necessary for both diagnostic approaches. Therefore, a total of 268 samples were analyzed by the previously validated equine-optimized porcine-specific insulin ELISA and another commonly used human-specific IRMA with particular attention being paid to the presence of endogenous equine insulin during the OGT procedure (n = 117 samples) and mainly exogenous non-equine insulin during the CGIT procedure (n = 151 samples). Insulin concentrations measured by the equine-optimized porcine-specific ELISA and the human-specific IRMA differed significantly in samples from both diagnostic procedures. In addition to marked differences in absolute insulin concentrations between both methods, they showed strong correlation. However, a Bland-Altman analysis indicated that the equine-optimized porcine-specific ELISA was, on average, 40.94 ± 35.20 µIU/mL lower than the human-specific IRMA in samples obtained from the OGT procedure and 90.82 ± 120 µIU/mL lower than the human-specific IRMA in samples obtained from CGIT procedure, both with the presence of proportional error. These findings suggest that results between the assays should not be considered interchangeable. The presence of exogenous insulin in samples obtained from IV testing for IR might especially attribute to the variable outcome of sample analyses with different immunoassays due to potential cross-reactivity of the exogenous insulin molecules or analogues with the assays' antibodies.

Summing up: Insulin concentrations measured by different methods need to be interpreted carefully in terms of making a clinical decision or diagnosis. Insulin concentrations obtained as results of basal or dynamic testing should be interpreted considering the immunoassay used for the quantification of the equine insulin. This research project provides a compilation of different immunoassay comparisons with provision of data for the conversion of insulin concentrations supplied by different immunoassays and for the transformation of previously defined reference ranges between immunoassays. In view of the large number of different test protocols which have been published and described, and missing consent regarding a global standardized diagnostic approach and harmonization of quantification of equine insulin, a comparison of immunoassays at least allows rough statements on test results. Furthermore, the results of this research project clearly indicate the strength and weaknesses in combining a specific diagnostic protocol with a specific immunoassay method and highlights the potential positive increase or negative decrease of the tests' diagnostic value based on the immunoassay-specific characteristics.

12 ZUSAMMENFASSUNG

Tobias Warnken

Vergleichende Untersuchungen zur labordiagnostischen Bestimmung von equinem Insulin unter Berücksichtigung der praxisrelevanten Anforderungen zur Diagnostik einer Insulindysregulation

Das Equine Metabolische Syndrome (EMS) ist eine heutzutage zunehmend häufiger auftretende Endokrinopathie und stellt ein großes Gesundheitsrisiko in der Pferdepopulation dar. Aktuelle Untersuchungen zeigen, dass neben der Vielzahl an teilweise charakteristischen klinischen Symptome des EMS, die Insulindysregulation (ID) mit einer einhergehenden Hyperinsulinämie das einzige Symptom ist, das eindeutig mit der Entstehung einer endokrinopathischen Hufrehe in Verbindung zu bringen ist. Eine ID kann sich auf verschiedene Arten manifestieren, zum Beispiel als basale Hyperinsulinämie, als übermäßige oder anhaltende hyperinsulinämische Reaktion auf oral aufgenommene oder intravenös verabreichte Kohlenhydrate oder als Insulinresistenz (IR) der peripheren Gewebe.

Die Diagnostik einer ID unter Feldbedingungen kann aufwendig, zeitintensiv und kostspielig sein. Sie kann unter Verwendung von basalen Blutproben oder auf der Grundlage von verschiedenen dynamischen Stimulationstests durchgeführt werden. Die unterschiedlichen Testverfahren zielen hierbei entweder auf die Identifizierung der ID oder einer IR ab. Gegenwärtig werden orale glykämische Stimulationstests empfohlen um eine ID durch eine unter standardisierten Bedingungen hervorgerufene postprandiale Hyperinsulinämie zu identifizieren. Unabhängig von den verschiedenen physiologischen Abläufen, die durch die verschiedenen Testverfahren hervorgerufen werden und deren unterschiedliche Aussagekraft in Bezug auf die Feststellung einer ID oder IR erfordern die meisten Diagnostikverfahren eine sich anschließende labordiagnostische Analyse der Insulinkonzentrationen in entnommenen Blutproben des untersuchten Patienten. Es zeigte sich jedoch bereits in früheren Studien, dass, zum Teil abhängig vom jeweiligen eingesetztem Immunoassay, deutliche Unterschiede zwischen den verschiedenen eingesetzten Methoden in Bezug auf die gemessenen Insulinkonzentrationen bestehen. Die meisten in der Veterinärmedizin verwendeten Immunoassays wurden ursprünglich für den Einsatz in der humanmedizinischen Labordiagnostik entwickelt und basieren auf Antikörpern, die gegen das humane Insulinmolekül gerichtet sind. Es ist jedoch bekannt, dass trotz weitreichender Sequenzhomologie unter den Vertebraten, Unterschiede in der Aminosäuresequenz zwischen dem equinen und dem humanen Insulin vorliegen.

Das Hauptziel dieses Forschungsprojekts bestand daher darin, die Quantifizierung von equinem Insulin unter der Berücksichtigung der klinischen Anforderungen und Bedingungen zu untersuchen und die Diagnostik der equinen ID durch eine geeignete Kombination aus einem dynamischen Diagnostiktest und der anschließenden Quantifizierung von equinem Insulin mittels einer geeigneten und zuverlässigen immunoassay-basierten Messmethode zu optimieren.

Das Ziel des ersten Teils dieses Forschungsprojekts war es, drei häufig verwendete Immunoassays im Hinblick auf ihre Eignung zur Analyse von equinem Insulin zu vergleichen. Besonderes Augenmerk wurde hierbei auf die Assay-spezifischen Eigenschaften und deren klinischer Anwendbarkeit bei der Beurteilung der ID gelegt. Im Rahmen dieser Untersuchungen wurden sowohl basale, nüchtern Blutproben, als auch unter Stimulation entnommene Blutproben untersucht. Mittels eines oralen Glukosetests (OGT) basierend auf der Applikation einer definierten Glukosemenge von 1g/kg Körpergewicht über eine Nasenschlundsonde konnte ein breites Spektrum an Proben mit unterschiedlichen Insulinkonzentrationen generiert werden.

Im Rahmen des ersten Teils des Forschungsprojektes wurden ein für den Einsatz beim Pferd optimierter Enzym-gebundener Immunosorbens-Assay (ELISA) basierend auf spezifischen gegen das porzine Insulin gerichteten Antikörpern, ein Radioimmunoassay (RIA), ebenfalls basierend auf spezifischen Antikörpern gegen das porzine Insulin und ein human-spezifischer Insulin Chemilumineszenz-Immunoassay (CLIA) verglichen. Alle drei verwendeten Immunoassays werden derzeit häufig und routinemäßig zur Messung von equinem Insulin in verschiedenen veterinärmedizinischen Laboren verwendet. Die Insulinkonzentrationen der basalen Blutproben unterschieden sich signifikant unter den drei verschiedenen Immunoassays. Die Analysen der während des OGT entnommenen Blutproben mit vergleichsweise höheren Insulinkonzentrationen ergaben signifikant niedrigere Insulinkonzentrationen im humanspezifischen CLIA im Vergleich zu dem für Pferde optimierten, für porzines Insulin spezifischen ELISA. Zusammenfassend zeigten sich große Diskrepanzen in Bezug auf die gemessenen Insulinkonzentrationen zwischen den drei verschiedenen Immunoassays, so dass diese sorgfältig interpretiert werden sollten. Die Ergebnisse der Untersuchung zeigen, dass die Berücksichtigung des zur Messung eingesetzten Immunoassays und die Anwendung zuverlässiger Assay-spezifischer Referenzbereiche oder Grenzwerte für die klinische Interpretation und Diagnose einer ID von besonderer Bedeutung und zwingend erforderlich sind.

Basierend auf diesen Erkenntnissen wurde das Ziel des zweiten Teils dieses Forschungsprojekts formuliert. Ziel war es, die Variationen der Insulinreaktionen auf einen OGT mittels Glukosverabreichung per Nasenschlundsonde in einer großen Kohorte von Pferden und Ponies weiter zu beschreiben und einen klinisch anwendbaren Grenzwert für die Bewertung einer ID bei der Quantifizierung des equinen Insulins mit Hilfe des zuvor validierten und für Pferde optimierten Insulin ELISA zu generieren. Hierfür wurden die Verläufe der Insulinkonzentrationen von 56 Pferden und Ponies nach einem standard-dosiertem OGT retrospektiv analysiert. Aufgrund der Tatsache, dass die anfängliche Datenvisualisierung keine klare Trennung von insulinsensitiven und insulin-dysregulierten Pferden ermöglichte, wurde eine modellbasierte Clustering-Methode verwendet, um die Verwendung einer willkürlichen Grenze für die Kategorisierung zu umgehen. Diese Methode berücksichtigte den individuellen Verlauf der endogenen Insulinkonzentration während des OGT und war in der Lage zwei verschiedene Cluster von Tieren zu identifizieren. Ein Cluster mit konstant niedrigen und ein Cluster mit signifikant höheren Insulinkonzentrationen als Reaktion auf die verabreichte Glukose während des OGT. Die Gruppe an Tieren mit niedrigen Insulinreaktionen wurde unabhängig von den Initialisierungsparametern des Algorithmus konsistent detektiert. Basierend auf dem 97,5% Quantil der Insulinkonzentrationen in diesem Cluster wurde ein

Grenzwert von 110 µIu/ml nach 120 Minuten berechnet. Somit wurde im Rahmen dieser Untersuchungen der erste Cut-off-Wert als Grundlage für die Diagnose einer ID bei Pferden basierend auf dem OGT-Verfahren und anschließender Bestimmung der Insulinkonzentration mit dem beschriebenen ELISA erarbeitet.

Da die Diagnostik einer ID jedoch auch auf der Beurteilung einer IR als einem Teilaspekt der ID beruhen kann, wurde ein drittes Forschungsprojekt durchgeführt. Der dritte Teil dieses Forschungsprojekts untersuchte den Einfluss von Insulinmessungen mit zwei verschiedenen Immunoassays in Proben die während eines OGT-Verfahrens zur Diagnostik einer ID entnommen wurden und in Proben die während eines kombinierten Glucose-Insulin-Tests (CGIT) zur Beurteilung der peripheren IR entnommen wurden. Trotz der unterschiedlichen zugrundeliegenden Testmechanismen und physiologischen Merkmale der beiden Testverfahren ist letztendlich die Quantifizierung von Insulin in beiden diagnostischen Ansätzen erforderlich. Im Rahmen dieser Untersuchungen wurden insgesamt 268 Proben durch den bereits im ersten und zweiten Teil des Forschungsprojektes verwendeten und validierten Insulin ELISA und einem anderen häufig verwendeten human-spezifischen immunradiometrische Assay (IRMA) analysiert. Besonders das Vorhandensein von endogenem equinem Insulin während des OGT-Verfahrens (n = 117 Proben) und des hauptsächlich vorhandenen exogenen Insulins während des CGIT-Verfahrens (n = 151 Proben) wurde in dieser Untersuchung genutzt um die Eignung der Immunoassays für den Einsatz in Kombination mit der jeweiligen Diagnostik zu untersuchen. Die Insulinkonzentrationen beider Messverfahren unterschieden sich in den Proben beider Testverfahren signifikant, zeigten jedoch eine enge positive Korrelation. Die Insulinkonzentrationen des für den Einsatz beim Pferd optimierten ELISA waren in den während des OGT entnommenen Proben durchschnittlich um 40,94 ± 35,20 µIu/ml niedriger im Vergleich zu dem human-spezifischen IRMA. In den Proben aus dem CGIT Verfahren ergab sich, dass der ELISA im Schnitt um 90,82 ± 120 µIu/ml niedrigere Insulinkonzentrationen ausgab als der human-spezifische IRMA. Zusätzlich zeigte sich auch hier ein proportionaler zunehmender Unterschied bei steigender Insulinkonzentration zwischen den beiden Methoden. Die Ergebnisse dieser Untersuchung legen wiederholt nahe, dass die

Ergebnisse zwischen diesen beiden Immunoassays ebenfalls nicht als austauschbar angesehen werden sollten. Insbesondere das Vorhandensein von exogenem Insulin in Proben aus intravenösen Diagnostiktests zur Abklärung einer IR, kann das Ergebnis aufgrund von Kreuzreaktivitäten zwischen den Antikörpern des Immunoassays und den vorhandenen exogenen Insulinmolekülen oder vorhandenen Insulinanaloga beeinflussen.

Zusammenfassend zeigen die hier vorliegenden Untersuchungen, dass Insulinkonzentrationen, die mit verschiedenen Methoden gemessen werden, sorgsam unter Berücksichtigung des verwendeten Immunoassays interpretiert werden sollten. Dies gilt sowohl für basale Blutproben zur nüchtern Bestimmung von equinem Insulin, als auch für Proben die während verschiedener Diagnostiktest entnommen werden. Nur so ist das sichere Stellen der Diagnose einer ID möglich und entsprechende therapeutische Maßnahmen abzuleiten.

Dieses Forschungsprojekt bietet eine Zusammenstellung und kritische Betrachtung verschiedener sich im veterinärmedizinischen Einsatz befindlicher Immunoassays unter Berücksichtigung der speziellen Anforderungen zur Diagnostik einer equinen ID. Die angestellten Vergleiche verschiedener Immunoassays ermöglichen aufgrund der zugrundliegenden Daten eine grobe Umrechnung von Insulinkonzentrationen aus verschiedenen Immunoassays. Dies ermöglicht zum einen die Transformation von zuvor definierten Referenzbereichen zwischen verschiedenen Immunoassays und erleichtert so den Einsatz verschiedener Tests und Immunoassays in der Praxis. Außerdem ermöglichen die durchgeführten Vergleichsuntersuchungen Vergleiche zwischen Ergebnissen verschiedener bereits publizierter Studien. Angesichts der Vielzahl der beschriebenen unterschiedlichen Diagnostikprotokolle, dem fehlenden Konsens zu einem weltweit standardisierten diagnostischen Ansatz sowie einer Harmonisierung der Bestimmung von equinem Insulin erlaubt der hier vorgenommene Vergleich von Immunoassays zumindest grobe Aussagen in Bezug auf die Testergebnisse aus verschiedenen Immunoassays. Darüber hinaus zeigen die Ergebnisse dieser Studie deutlich die unterschiedlichen Stärken und Schwächen der Kombination eines bestimmten diagnostischen Testverfahrens und einem bestimmten Immunoassays und verdeutlichen die potenzielle positive oder negative

Zunahme des diagnostischen Testwerts auf der Grundlage der immunoassay-spezifischen Eigenschaften der Insulinanalytik.

13 REFERENCES

Andreasson U., Perret-Liaudet A., Van Waalwijk Van Doorn L. J. C., Blennow K., Chiasserini D., Engelborghs S., Fladby T., Genc S., Kruse N., Kuiperij H. B., Kulic L., Lewczuk P., Mollenhauer B., Mroczko B., Parnetti L., Vanmechelen E., Verbeek M. M., Winblad B., Zetterberg H., Koel-Simmelink M. and Teunissen C. E. (2015) A Practical Guide to Immunoassay Method Validation. Frontiers in neurology, 179–179

Anderson L. and Hunter C. L. (2006) Quantitative mass spectrometric multiple reaction monitoring assays for major plasma proteins. Mol Cell Proteomics, 4, 573–588

American Society For Veterinary Clinical Pathology (ASCCP) – Arnold J., Barnhart K., Blanco J., Davies R., Davis D., Flatland B., Freeman K., Friedrichs K., Gunn-Christie R., Harr K., Kocmarek H., Korcal D. Matthews J., Messick J., Pearson R., Pedersen S., Ruotsala K., Shanahan L., Szladovits B., Vap L., (2009) Principles of Quality Assurance and Standards for Veterinary Clinical Pathology – American Clinical Veterinary Pathology Annual Meeting. http://www.asvcp.org/pubs/pdf/ASVCPQualityControlGuidelines.pdf. Accessed 31 Jan 2018.

Asplin K. E., Patterson-Kane J. C., Sillence M. N., Pollitt C. C. and McGowan C. M. (2010) Histopathology of insulin-induced laminitis in ponies. Equine Vet J, 8, 700–706

Asplin K. E., Sillence M. N., Pollitt C. C. and McGowan C. M. (2007) Induction of laminitis by prolonged hyperinsulinaemia in clinically normal ponies. Vet J, 3, 530–535

Aydin S. (2015) A short history, principles, and types of ELISA, and our laboratory experience with peptide/protein analyses using ELISA. Peptides, 72, 4–15

Azim, M. A., Hasan, M., Ansari, I., & Nasreen, F. (2018). Chemiluminescence Immunoassay: Basic Mechanism and Applications. Bangladesh J. Nucl. Med, 18(2), 171–178

Babson (2013) IMMULITE® and IMMULITE 1000. In Wild D. (Ed): The Immunoassay Handbook: Theory and Applications of Ligand Binding, ELISA and Related Techniques. 4th Edition, Elsevier Science, Newnes, 571–574

Babson (2013) IMMULITE® 2000 and IMMULITE 2000xpi. In Wild D. (Ed): The Immunoassay Handbook: Theory and Applications of Ligand Binding, ELISA and Related Techniques. 4th Edition, Elsevier Science, Newnes, 575–578

Bailey S. R., Habershon-Butcher J. L., Ransom K. J., Elliott J. and Menzies-Gow N. J. (2008) Hypertension and insulin resistance in a mixed-breed population of ponies predisposed to laminitis. Am J Vet Res, 1, 122–129

Bailey S. R., Menzies-Gow N. J., Harris P. A., Habershon-Butcher J. L., Crawford C., Berhane Y., Boston R. C. and Elliott J. (2007) Effect of dietary fructans and dexamethasone administration on the insulin response of ponies predisposed to laminitis. J Am Vet Med Assoc, 9, 1365–1373

Bamford N. J., Baskerville C. L., Harris P. A. and Bailey S. R. (2015) Postprandial glucose, insulin, and glucagon-like peptide-1 responses of different equine breeds adapted to meals containing micronized maize. Journal of Animal Science, 7, 3377–3383

Bamford N. J., Potter S. J., Harris P. A. and Bailey S. R. (2014) Breed differences in insulin sensitivity and insulinemic responses to oral glucose in horses and ponies of moderate body condition score. Domest Anim Endocrinol, 47, 101–107

Banse H. E., McCann J., Yang F., Wagg C. and Mcfarlane D. (2014) Comparison of two methods for measurement of equine insulin. J Vet Diagn Invest, 4, 527–530

Banse H. E. and McFarlane D. (2014) Comparison of Three Methods for Evaluation of Equine Insulin Regulation in Horses of Varied Body Condition Score. J Equine Vet Sci, 6, 742–748

Berg J. M., Tymoczko J. L., Gatto G.J., Stryer L., Held A., Held M. (2018) Stryer Biochemie. 8th Edition. Springer Spektrum, Berlin

Bertin F. R. and De Laat M. A. (2017) The diagnosis of equine insulin dysregulation. Equine Vet J, 5, 570–576

Bertin F. R. and Sojka-Kritchevsky J. E. (2013) Comparison of a 2-step insulin-response test to conventional insulin-sensitivity testing in horses. Domest Anim Endocrinol, 1, 19–25

Borer-Weir K. E., Bailey S. R., Menzies-Gow N. J., Harris P. A. and Elliott J. (2012) Evaluation of a commercially available radioimmunoassay and species-specific ELISAs for measurement of high concentrations of insulin in equine serum. Am J Vet Res, 10, 1596–1602

Caltabilota T. J., Earl L. R., Thompson D. L., Jr., Clavier S. E. and Mitcham P. B. (2010) Hyperleptinemia in mares and geldings: assessment of insulin sensitivity from glucose responses to insulin injection. J Anim Sci, 9, 2940–2949

Cantarelli C., Dau S. L., Stefanello S., Azevedo M. S., De Bastiani G. R., Palma H. E., Brass K. E. and De La Côrte F. D. (2018) Evaluation of oral sugar test response for detection of equine metabolic syndrome in obese Crioulo horses. Domest Anim Endocrinol, 63, 31–37

Carslake H. B., Pinchbeck G. L. and McGowan C. M. (2017) Evaluation of a Chemiluminescent Immunoassay for Measurement of Equine Insulin. J Vet Intern Med, 2, 568–574

Carter R. A., Treiber K. H., Geor R. J., Douglass L. and Harris P. A. (2009) Prediction of incipient pasture-associated laminitis from hyperinsulinaemia, hyperleptinaemia and generalised and localised obesity in a cohort of ponies. Equine Vet J, 2, 171–178

Cartmill J. A., Thompson D. L., Jr., Storer W. A., Gentry L. R. and Huff N. K. (2003) Endocrine responses in mares and geldings with high body condition scores grouped by high vs. low resting leptin concentrations. J Anim Sci, 9, 2311–2321

Chameroy K. A., Frank N., Elliott S. B. and Boston R. C. (2016) Comparison of Plasma Active Glucagon-Like Peptide 1 Concentrations in Normal Horses and Those With Equine Metabolic Syndrome and in Horses Placed on a High-Grain Diet. J Equine Vet Sci, 40, 16–25

Chen Z., Caulfield M. P., McPhaul M. J., Reitz R. E., Taylor S. W. and Clarke N. J. (2013) Quantitative insulin analysis using liquid chromatography-tandem mass spectrometry in a high-throughput clinical laboratory. Clin Chem, 9, 1349–1356

Christenson R. H. and Duh S. H. (2012) Methodological and Analytic Considerations for Blood Biomarkers. Prog Cardiovasc Dis, 1, 25–33

Clinical and Laboratory Standards Institute (2008) Defining, Establishing, and Verifying Reference Intervals in the Clinical Laboratory; Approved Guideline. 3rd Edition, Wayne

Conlon J. M. (2001) Evolution of the insulin molecule: insights into structure-activity and phylogenetic relationships. Peptides, 7, 1183–1193

Davies C. (2013) Principles of competitive and immunometric assays (including ELISA). In Wild D. (Ed): The Immunoassay Handbook: Theory and Applications of

Ligand Binding, ELISA and Related Techniques. 4th Edition, Elsevier Science, Newnes, 29–60

Davies C. (2013) Immunoassay performance measures. In Wild D. (Ed): The Immunoassay Handbook: Theory and Applications of Ligand Binding, ELISA and Related Techniques. 4th Edition, Elsevier Science, Newnes, 11–28

Dayaldasani A., Rodríguez Espinosa M., Ocón Sánchez P. and Pérez Valero V. (2015) Cross-reactivity of insulin analogues with three insulin assays. Ann Clin Biochem, 3, 312–318

De Graaf-Roelfsema E. (2014) Glucose homeostasis and the enteroinsular axis in the horse: A possible role in equine metabolic syndrome. Vet J, 1, 11–18

De Koster J. D. and Opsomer G. (2013) Insulin resistance in dairy cows. Vet Clin North Am Food Anim Pract, 2, 299–322

De Laat M. A. (2019) Science in brief: Progress in endocrinopathic laminitis research: Have we got a foothold? Equine Vet J, 2, 141–142

De Laat M. A., McGowan C. M., Sillence M. N. and Pollitt C. C. (2010) Equine laminitis: induced by 48 h hyperinsulinaemia in Standardbred horses. Equine Vet J, 2, 129–135

De Laat M. A., McGree J. M. and Sillence M. N. (2016a) Equine hyperinsulinemia: investigation of the enteroinsular axis during insulin dysregulation. Am J Physiol Endocrinol Metab, 1, E61–72

De Laat M. A. and Sillence M. N. (2017) The repeatability of an oral glucose test in ponies. Equine Vet J, 2, 238–243

De Laat M. A., Sillence M. N., McGowan C. M. and Pollitt C. C. (2012) Continuous intravenous infusion of glucose induces endogenous hyperinsulinaemia and lamellar histopathology in Standardbred horses. Vet J, 3, 317–322

De Laat M. A., Sillence M. N. and Reiche D. B. (2019) Phenotypic, hormonal, and clinical characteristics of equine endocrinopathic laminitis. J Vet Intern Med, 3, 1456–1463

De Laat M. A., Van Haeften J. J. and Sillence M. N. (2016b) The effect of oral and intravenous dextrose on C-peptide secretion in ponies. J Anim Sci, 2, 574–580

Dimeski G. (2008) Interference testing. Clin Biochem Rev, S43–48

Divers T. J. (2008) Endocrine Testing in Horses: Metabolic Syndrome and Cushing's Disease. J Equine Vet Sci, 5, 315–316

Donaldson M. T., Jorgensen A. J. and Beech J. (2004) Evaluation of suspected pituitary pars intermedia dysfunction in horses with laminitis. J Am Vet Med Assoc, 7, 1123–1127

Dudley R. F. (1990) Chemiluminescence Immunoassay: An Alternative to RIA. Lab Med, 4, 216–222

Duehlmeier R., Deegen E., Fuhrmann H., Widdel A. and Sallmann H. P. (2001) Glucose-dependent insulinotropic polypeptide (GIP) and the enteroinsular axis in equines (Equus caballus). Comp Biochem Physiol A Mol Integr Physiol, 2–3, 563–575

Dunbar L. K., Mielnicki K. A., Dembek K. A., Toribio R. E. and Burns T. A. (2016) Evaluation of Four Diagnostic Tests for Insulin Dysregulation in Adult Light-Breed Horses. J Vet Intern Med, 3, 885–891

Durham A. E., Frank N., McGowan C. M., Menzies-Gow N. J., Roelfsema E., Vervuert I., Feige K. and Fey K. (2019) ECEIM consensus statement on equine metabolic syndrome. J Vet Intern Med, 2, 335–349

Durham A. E., Hughes K. J., Cottle H. J., Rendle D. I. and Boston R. C. (2009) Type 2 diabetes mellitus with pancreatic β cell dysfunction in 3 horses confirmed with minimal model analysis. Equine Vet J, 9, 924–929

Eiler H., Frank N., Andrews F. M., Oliver J. W. and Fecteau K. A. (2005) Physiologic assessment of blood glucose homeostasis via combined intravenous glucose and insulin testing in horses. Am J Vet Res, 9, 1598–1604

Engvall E. (2010) The ELISA, enzyme-linked immunosorbent assay. Clin Chem, 2, 319–320

Engvall E, Perlmann P. Enzyme-linked immunosorbent assay (ELISA). Quantitative assay of immunoglobulin G. Immunochemistry 1971, 8, 871–4

Equine Endocrinology Group – Frank N., Bailey S., Bertin F. R., Burns T., De Laat M., Durham A., Kritchevsky J., Menzies-Gow N., Tadros L. (2018) Recommendations for the diagnosis and treatment of Equine Metabolic Syndrome (EMS). https://sites.tufts.edu/equineendogroup/files/2018/09/2018-Final-EMS_Recommendations_Web.pdf. Accessed 05 Nov 2018.

Equine Endocrinology Group – Schott H., Andrews F., Durham A., Frank N., Hart K., Kritchevsky J., McFarlane D., Tadros L. (2017) Recommendations for the Diagnosis and Treatment of Pituitary Pars Intermedia Dysfunction (PPID). https://sites.tufts.edu/equineendogroup/files/2017/11/2017-EEG-Recommendations-PPID.pdf. Accessed 12 Nov 2018.

Findlay J. W. A., Smith W. C., Lee J. W., Nordblom G. D., Das I., Desilva B. S., Khan M. N. and Bowsher R. R. (2000) Validation of immunoassays for bioanalysis: a pharmaceutical industry perspective. J Pharm Biomed Anal, 6, 1249–1273

Fitzgerald D. M., Anderson S. T., Sillence M. N. and De Laat M. A. (2019a) The cresty neck score is an independent predictor of insulin dysregulation in ponies. PLoS One, 7, e0220203

Fitzgerald D. M., Walsh D. M., Sillence M. N., Pollitt C. C. and De Laat M. A. (2019b) Insulin and incretin responses to grazing in insulin-dysregulated and healthy ponies. J Vet Intern Med, 1, 225–232

Fowden A. L., Comline R. S. and Silver M. (1984) Insulin secretion and carbohydrate metabolism during pregnancy in the mare. Equine Vet J, 4, 239–246

Frank N. (2011) Equine metabolic syndrome. Vet Clin North Am Equine Pract, 1, 73–92

Frank N., Elliott S. B., Brandt L. E. and Keisler D. H. (2006) Physical characteristics, blood hormone concentrations, and plasma lipid concentrations in obese horses with insulin resistance. J Am Vet Med Assoc, 9, 1383–1390

Frank N. and Geor R. (2014) Current best practice in clinical management of equine endocrine patients. Equine Vet Educ, 1, 6–9

Frank N., Geor R. J., Bailey S. R., Durham A. E., Johnson P. J. and American College of Veterinary Internal M. (2010) Equine metabolic syndrome. J Vet Intern Med, 3, 467–475

Frank N. and Tadros E. M. (2014) Insulin dysregulation. Equine Vet J, 1, 103–112

Freestone J. F., Wolfsheimer K. J., Kamerling S. G., Church G., Hamra J. and Bagwell C. (1991) Exercise induced hormonal and metabolic changes in Thoroughbred horses: effects of conditioning and acepromazine. Equine Vet J, 3, 219–223

Friemel H. (1991) Immunelektrophorese. In Friemel H. (Ed): Immunologische Arbeitsmethoden. 4th Edition, Gustav Fischer Verlag, Jena, 98–187

Galey F. D., Whiteley H. E., Goetz T. E., Kuenstler A. R., Davis C. A. and Beasley V. R. (1991) Black-Walnut (Juglans-Nigra) Toxicosis – a Model for Equine Laminitis. J Comp Pathol, 3, 313–326

Garcia M. C. and Beech J. (1986) Equine intravenous glucose tolerance test: glucose and insulin responses of healthy horses fed grain or hay and of horses with pituitary adenoma. Am J Vet Res, 3, 570–572

Garner H. E., Coffman J. R., Hahn A. W., Hutcheson D. P. and Tumbleson M. E. (1975) Equine Laminitis of Alimentary Origin – Experimental Model. Am J Vet Res, 4, 441–444

Geffre A., Friedrichs K., Harr K., Concordet D., Trumel C. and Braun J. P. (2009) Reference values: a review. Vet Clin Pathol, 3, 288–298

Giles S. L., Nicol C. J., Rands S. A. and Harris P. A. (2015) Assessing the seasonal prevalence and risk factors for nuchal crest adiposity in domestic horses and ponies using the Cresty Neck Score. BMC Vet Res, 13

Giles S. L., Rands S. A., Nicol C. J. and Harris P. A. (2014) Obesity prevalence and associated risk factors in outdoor living domestic horses and ponies. PeerJ, e299

Giraudi G., Anfossi L., Rosso I., Baggiani C., Giovannoli C. and Tozzi C. (1999) A General Method To Perform a Noncompetitive Immunoassay for Small Molecules. Anal Chem, 20, 4697–4700

Goldsmith S. J. (1975) Radioimmunoassay: Review of basic principles. Semin Nucl Med, 2, 125–152

Haddad R. A., Giacherio D. and Barkan A. L. (2019) Interpretation of common endocrine laboratory tests: technical pitfalls, their mechanisms and practical considerations. Clinical Diabetes and Endocrinology, 1, 12

Haeckel R. and Wosniok W. (2004) The discordance rate, a new concept for combining diagnostic decisions with analytical performance characteristics. 2. Defining analytical goals applied to the diagnosis of type 2 diabetes by blood glucose concentrations. Clin Chem Lab Med, 2, 198–203

Heliczer N., Gerber V., Bruckmaier R., Van Der Kolk J. H. and De Solis C. N. (2017) Cardiovascular findings in ponies with equine metabolic syndrome. J Amer Vet Med Assn, 9, 1027–1035

Ho E. N., Wan T. S., Wong A. S., Lam K. K. and Stewart B. D. (2008) Doping control analysis of insulin and its analogues in equine plasma by liquid chromatography-tandem mass spectrometry. J Chromatogr A, 2, 183–190

Ho E. N., Wan T. S., Wong A. S., Lam K. K. and Stewart B. D. (2011) Doping control analysis of insulin and its analogues in equine urine by liquid chromatography-tandem mass spectrometry. J Chromatogr A, 8, 1139–1146

Hoffman R. M., Boston R. C., Stefanovski D., Kronfeld D. S. and Harris P. A. (2003) Obesity and diet affect glucose dynamics and insulin sensitivity in Thoroughbred geldings. J Anim Sci, 9, 2333–2342

International Organization for Standardization (1994) ISO 5725-1. Accuracy (trueness and precision) of measurement methods and results – Part 1: General principles and definitions. https://www.iso.org/obp/ui/#iso:std:iso:5725:-1:ed-1:v1:en. Assessed 15 April 2019.

Iversen L., Jensen A. L., Høier R. and Aaes H. (1999) Biological Variation of Canine Serum Thyrotropin (TSH) Concentration. Vet Clin Path, 1, 16–19

Jacob S. I., Geor R. J., Weber P. S. D., Harris P. A. and McCue M. E. (2018a) Effect of age and dietary carbohydrate profiles on glucose and insulin dynamics in horses. Equine Vet J, 2, 249–254

Jacob S. I., Murray K. J., Rendahl A. K., Geor R. J., Schultz N. E. and McCue M. E. (2018b) Metabolic perturbations in Welsh Ponies with insulin dysregulation, obesity, and laminitis. J Vet Intern Med, 3, 1215–1233

Jandreski M. A. (1998) Chemiluminescence technology in immunoassays. Lab Med, 9, 555–560

Jensen A. L. and Kjelgaard-Hansen M. (2006) Method comparison in the clinical laboratory. Vet Clin Path, 3, 276–286

Jocelyn N. A., Harris P. A. and Menzies-Gow N. J. (2018) Effect of varying the dose of corn syrup on the insulin and glucose response to the oral sugar test. Equine Vet J, 6, 836–841

Johnson P. J. (2002) The equine metabolic syndrome peripheral Cushing's syndrome. Vet Clin North Am Equine Pract, 2, 271–293

Kahn C. R. (1978) Insulin resistance, insulin insensitivity, and insulin unresponsiveness: a necessary distinction. Metabolism, 12 Suppl 2, 1893–1902

Kahn C. R. (1980) Role of insulin receptors in insulin-resistant states. Metabolism, 5, 455–466

Karikoski N. P., Horn I., Mcgowan T. W. and McGowan C. M. (2011) The prevalence of endocrinopathic laminitis among horses presented for laminitis at a first-opinion/referral equine hospital. Domest Anim Endocrinol, 3, 111–117

Kenez A., Warnken T., Feige K. and Huber K. (2018) Lower plasma trans-4-hydroxyproline and methionine sulfoxide levels are associated with insulin dysregulation in horses. BMC Vet Res, 1, 146

Koeller G., Bassewitz K. and Schusser G. F. (2016) Reference ranges of insulin, insulin like growth factor-1 and adrenocorticotropic hormone in ponies. Tierarztl Prax Ausg G Grosstiere Nutztiere, 1, 19–25

Kricka L. J. (1991) Chemiluminescent and bioluminescent techniques. Clin Chem, 9, 1472–1481

Kronfeld D. S., Treiber K. H. and Geor R. J. (2005) Comparison of nonspecific indications and quantitative methods for the assessment of insulin resistance in horses and ponies. J Am Vet Med Assoc, 5, 712–719

Kunkel S. (1991) Radiometrische Verfahren. In Friemel H. (Ed): Immunologische Arbeitsmethoden. 4th Edition, Gustav Fischer Verlag, Jena, 120 – 134

Kuuranne T., Thomas A., Leinonen A., Delahaut P., Bosseloir A., Schanzer W. and Thevis M. (2008) Insulins in equine urine: qualitative analysis by immunoaffinity purification and liquid chromatography/tandem mass spectrometry for doping control purposes in horse-racing. Rapid Commun Mass Spectrom, 3, 355–362

Lee J. W., Devanarayan V., Barrett Y. C., Weiner R., Allinson J., Fountain S., Keller S., Weinryb I., Green M., Duan L., Rogers J. A., Millham R., O'brien P. J., Sailstad J., Khan M., Ray C. and Wagner J. A. (2006) Fit-for-purpose method development and validation for successful biomarker measurement. Pharm Res, 2, 312–328

Lequin R. M. (2005) Enzyme Immunoassay (EIA)/Enzyme-Linked Immunosorbent Assay (ELISA). Clin Chem, 12, 2415–2418

Lewis S. L., Holl H. M., Long M. T., Mallicote M. F. and Brooks S. A. (2018) Use of principle component analysis to quantitatively score the equine metabolic syndrome phenotype in an Arabian horse population. Plos One, 7, e0200583

Lewis S. L., Holl H. M., Streeter C., Posbergh C., Schanbacher B. J., Place N. J., Mallicote M. F., Long M. T. and Brooks S. A. (2017) Genomewide association study reveals a risk locus for equine metabolic syndrome in the Arabian horse. J Anim Sci, 3, 1071–1079

Liddell E. (2013) Antibodies. In Wild D. (Ed): The Immunoassay Handbook: Theory and Applications of Ligand Binding, ELISA and Related Techniques. 4th Edition, Elsevier Science, Newnes, 245–266

Lindase S., Nostell K. and Brojer J. (2016) A modified oral sugar test for evaluation of insulin and glucose dynamics in horses. Acta Vet Scand, Suppl 1, 64

Mair T. S., Hillyer M. H., Taylor F. G. and Pearson G. R. (1991) Small intestinal malabsorption in the horse: an assessment of the specificity of the oral glucose tolerance test. Equine Vet J, 5, 344–346

Manfredi J. M. (2016) Identifying breed differences in insulin dynamics, skeletal muscle and adipose tissue histology and biology. East Lansing, Michigan Stat University, Diss. vet. Med.

Marca M., Loste A., Orden I., González J. and Marsellá J. (2001) Evaluation of canine serum thyrotropin (TSH) concentration: comparison of three analytical procedures. J Vet Diagn Invest, 2, 106–110

Marcovina S., Bowsher R. R., Miller W. G., Staten M., Myers G., Caudill S. P., Campbell S. E. and Steffes M. W. (2007) Standardization of Insulin Immunoassays: Report of the American Diabetes Association Workgroup. Clin Chem, 4, 711–716

Maresh M. (2001) Diabetes in pregnancy. Curr Opin Obstet Gynecol, 2, 103–107

Marshall W. J. and Bangert S. K. (2008) Clinical biochemistry: metabolic and clinical aspects. 3rd Edition, Elsevier Health Sciences, Philadelphia, p. 19

Mastro L. M., Adams A. A. and Urschel K. L. (2015) Pituitary pars intermedia dysfunction does not necessarily impair insulin sensitivity in old horses. Domest Anim Endocrinol, 50, 14–25

McCue M. E., Geor R. J. and Schultz N. (2015) Equine Metabolic Syndrome: A Complex Disease Influenced by Genetics and the Environment. J Equine Vet Sci, 5, 367–375

McFarlane D. (2011) Equine pituitary pars intermedia dysfunction. Vet Clin North Am Equine Pract, 1, 93–113

McFarlane D. and Cribb A. E. (2005) Systemic and pituitary pars intermedia antioxidant capacity associated with pars intermedia oxidative stress and dysfunction in horses. Am J Vet Res, 12, 2065–2072

McGowan C. (2008) The Role of Insulin in Endocrinopathic Laminitis. J Equine Vet Sci, 10, 603–607

McGowan C. M. (2010) Endocrinopathic Laminitis. Vet Clin North Am Equine Pract, 2, 233–237

McGowan T. W., Pinchbeck G. P. and McGowan C. M. (2013) Prevalence, risk factors and clinical signs predictive for equine pituitary pars intermedia dysfunction in aged horses. Equine Vet J, 1, 74–79

Meier A., De Laat M., Reiche D., Fitzgerald D. and Sillence M. (2019) The efficacy and safety of velagliflozin over 16 weeks as a treatment for insulin dysregulation in ponies. BMC Vet Res, 1, 65

Meier A., Reiche D., De Laat M., Pollitt C., Walsh D. and Sillence M. (2018) The sodium-glucose co-transporter 2 inhibitor velagliflozin reduces hyperinsulinemia and prevents laminitis in insulin-dysregulated ponies. PLoS One, 9, e0203655

Meier A. D., De Laat M. A., Reiche D. B., Pollitt C. C., Walsh D. M., McGree J. M. and Sillence M. N. (2017) The oral glucose test predicts laminitis risk in ponies fed a diet high in nonstructural carbohydrates. Domest Anim Endocrinol, 63, 1–9

Meier J. J., Veldhuis J. D. and Butler P. C. (2005) Pulsatile insulin secretion dictates systemic insulin delivery by regulating hepatic insulin extraction in humans. Diabetes, 6, 1649–1656

Menzies-Gow N. J., Harris P. A. and Elliott J. (2017) Prospective cohort study evaluating risk factors for the development of pasture-associated laminitis in the United Kingdom. Equine Vet J, 3, 300–306

Metzar (2013) ADVIA Centaur® xp. In Wild D. (Ed): The Immunoassay Handbook: Theory and Applications of Ligand Binding, ELISA and Related Techniques. 4th Edition, Elsevier Science, Newnes, 567–570

Miller W. G., Thienpont L. M., Van Uytfanghe K., Clark P. M., Lindstedt P., Nilsson G. and Steffes M. W. (2009) Toward Standardization of Insulin Immunoassays. Clin Chem, 5, 1011–1018

Morgan R. A., McGowan T. W. and McGowan C. M. (2014) Prevalence and risk factors for hyperinsulinaemia in ponies in Queensland, Australia. Aust Vet J, 4, 101–106

Muniyappa R., Lee S., Chen H. and Quon M. J. (2008) Current approaches for assessing insulin sensitivity and resistance in vivo: advantages, limitations, and appropriate usage. Am J Physiol Endocrinol Metab, 1, E15–26

Norton E. M., Avila F., Schultz N. E., Mickelson J. R., Geor R. J. and Mccue M. E. (2019a) Evaluation of an HMGA2 variant for pleiotropic effects on height and metabolic traits in ponies. J Vet Intern Med, 2, 942–952

Norton E. M., Schultz N. E., Rendahl A. K., McFarlane D., Geor R. J., Mickelson J. R. and McCue M. E. (2019b) Heritability of metabolic traits associated with equine metabolic syndrome in Welsh ponies and Morgan horses. Equine Vet J, 4, 475–480

Öberg J., Bröjer J., Wattle O. and Lilliehöök I. (2011) Evaluation of an equine-optimized enzyme-linked immunosorbent assay for serum insulin measurement and stability study of equine serum insulin. Comp Clin Path, 6, 1291–1300

Olley R. B., Carslake H. B., Ireland J. L. and McGowan C. M. (2019) Comparison of fasted basal insulin with the combined glucose-insulin test in horses and ponies with suspected insulin dysregulation. Vet J, 105351

Owen W. E. and Roberts W. L. (2004) Cross-Reactivity of Three Recombinant Insulin Analogs with Five Commercial Insulin Immunoassays. Clin Chem, 1, 257–259

Patterson-Kane J. C., Karikoski N. P. and McGowan C. M. (2018) Paradigm shifts in understanding equine laminitis. Vet J, 231, 33–40

Piechotta M., Arndt M. and Hoppen H. O. (2010) Autoantibodies against thyroid hormones and their influence on thyroxine determination with chemiluminescence immunoassay in dogs. Journal of veterinary science, 3, 191–196

Pleasant R. S., Suagee J. K., Thatcher C. D., Elvinger F. and Geor R. J. (2013) Adiposity, plasma insulin, leptin, lipids, and oxidative stress in mature light breed horses. J Vet Intern Med, 3, 576–582

Pollitt C. (2004) Equine laminitis. Clin Tech Equine Pract, 3, 33–44

Pollitt C. C. (1996) Basement membrane pathology: A feature of acute equine laminitis. Equine Vet J, 1, 38–46

Pollitt C. C. and Visser M. B. (2010) Carbohydrate alimentary overload laminitis. Vet Clin North Am Equine Pract, 1, 65–78

Porstmann T. and Porstmann B. (1991) Enzymimmunoassay. In: Immunologische Arbeitsmethoden, H. Freimel, Eds; 4. Edition, Gustav Fischer Verlag, Jena, 135–187

Praither J. D. (1985) Basic Principles of Radioimmunoassay Testing: A Simple Approach. J Nuc Med Tech, 1, 34–43

Pratt-Phillips S. E., Geor R. J. and McCutcheon L. J. (2015) Comparison among the euglycemic-hyperinsulinemic clamp, insulin-modified frequently sampled intravenous glucose tolerance test, and oral glucose tolerance test for assessment of insulin sensitivity in healthy Standardbreds. Am J Vet Res, 1, 84–91

Pratt S. E., Geor R. J. and McCutcheon L. J. (2005) Repeatability of 2 methods for assessment of insulin sensitivity and glucose dynamics in horses. J Vet Intern Med, 6, 883–888

Rabkin R., Ryan M. P. and Duckworth W. C. (1984) The Renal Metabolism of Insulin. Diabetologia, 3, 351–357

Ralston S. L. (2002) Insulin and glucose regulation. Vet Clin North Am Equine Pract, 2, 295–304

Rijnen K. E. and Van Der Kolk J. H. (2003) Determination of reference range values indicative of glucose metabolism and insulin resistance by use of glucose clamp techniques in horses and ponies. Am J Vet Res, 10, 1260–1264

Saltiel A. R. and Kahn C. R. (2001) Insulin signalling and the regulation of glucose and lipid metabolism. Nature, 6865, 799–806

Schott H. C. (2002) Pituitary pars intermedia dysfunction: equine Cushing's disease. Vet Clin North Am Equine Pract, 2, 237–270

Schuver A., Frank N., Chameroy K. A. and Elliott S. B. (2014) Assessment of Insulin and Glucose Dynamics by Using an Oral Sugar Test in Horses. J Equine Vet Sci, 4, 465–470

Shanik M. H., Xu Y., Skrha J., Dankner R., Zick Y. and Roth J. (2008) Insulin resistance and hyperinsulinemia: is hyperinsulinemia the cart or the horse? Diabetes Care, S262–268

Skelley D. S., Brown L. P. and Besch P. K. (1973) Radioimmunoassay. Clin Chem, 2, 146–186

Smith S., Harris P. A. and Menzies-Gow N. J. (2016) Comparison of the in-feed glucose test and the oral sugar test. Equine Vet J, 2, 224–227

Stanczyk F. Z. and Clarke N. J. (2010) Advantages and challenges of mass spectrometry assays for steroid hormones. J Steroid Biochem Mol Biol, 3–5, 491–495

Staten M. A., Stern M. P., Miller W. G., Steffes M. W., Campbell S. E. and Insulin Standardization W. (2010) Insulin assay standardization: leading to measures of insulin sensitivity and secretion for practical clinical care. Diabetes care, 1, 205–206

Steiner D. F. (2004) The proinsulin C-peptide--a multirole model. Exp Diabesity Res, 1, 7–14

Stockl D., Dewitte K. and Thienpont L. M. (1998) Validity of linear regression in method comparison studies: is it limited by the statistical model or the quality of the analytical input data? Clin Chem, 11, 2340–2346

Stretton A. O. (2002) The first sequence. Fred Sanger and insulin. Genetics, 2, 527–532

Thatcher C. D., Pleasant R. S., Geor R. J., Elvinger F., Negrin K. A., Franklin J., Gay L. and Werre S. R. (2008) Prevalence of obesity in mature horses: an equine body condition study. J Anim Physiol Anim Nutr, 2, 222–222

Thevis M., Thomas A. and Schänzer W. (2011) Doping control analysis of selected peptide hormones using LC–MS(/MS). Forensic Sci Int, 1, 35–41

Thomas A., Schanzer W., Delahaut P. and Thevis M. (2009) Sensitive and fast identification of urinary human, synthetic and animal insulin by means of nano-UPLC coupled with high-resolution/high-accuracy mass spectrometry. Drug Test Anal, 5, 219–227

Tinworth K. D., Wynn P. C., Boston R. C., Harris P. A., Sillence M. N., Thevis M., Thomas A. and Noble G. K. (2011) Evaluation of commercially available assays for the measurement of equine insulin. Domest Anim Endocrinol, 2, 81–90

Tinworth K. D., Wynn P. C., Harris P. A., Sillence M. N. and Noble G. K. (2009) Optimising the Siemens Coat-A-Count Radioimmunoassay to Measure Insulin in Equine Plasma. J Equine Vet Sci, 5, 411–413

Toft-Nielsen M. B., Damholt M. B., Madsbad S., Hilsted L. M., Hughes T. E., Michelsen B. K. and Holst J. J. (2001a) Determinants of the impaired secretion of glucagon-like peptide-1 in type 2 diabetic patients. J Clin Endocrinol Metab, 8, 3717–3723

Toft-Nielsen M. B., Madsbad S. and Holst J. J. (2001b) Determinants of the effectiveness of glucagon-like peptide-1 in type 2 diabetes. J Clin Endocrinol Metab, 8, 3853–3860

Treiber K. H., Kronfeld D. S., Hess T. M., Boston R. C. and Harris P. A. (2005) Use of proxies and reference quintiles obtained from minimal model analysis for determination of insulin sensitivity and pancreatic beta-cell responsiveness in horses. Am J Vet Res, 12, 2114–2121

Treiber K. H., Kronfeld D. S., Hess T. M., Byrd B. M., Splan R. K. and Staniar W. B. (2006) Evaluation of genetic and metabolic predispositions and nutritional risk factors for pasture-associated laminitis in ponies. J Am Vet Med Assoc, 10, 1538–1545

Urschel K. L., Escobar J., McCutcheon L. J. and Geor R. J. (2014a) Effects of the rate of insulin infusion during isoglycemic, hyperinsulinemic clamp procedures on measures of insulin action in healthy, mature thoroughbred mares. Domest Anim Endocrinol, 47, 83–91

Urschel K. L., Escobar J., McCutcheon L. J. and Geor R. J. (2014b) Insulin infusion stimulates whole-body protein synthesis and activates the upstream and downstream effectors of mechanistic target of rapamycin signaling in the gluteus medius muscle of mature horses. Domest Anim Endocrinol, 47, 92–100

U.S. Department of Health and Human Services, Food and Drug Administration. Guidance for Industry. Bioanalytical Method Validation. http://www.fda.gov/Drugs/GuidanceComplianceRegulatoryInformation/Guidances/default.htm. Accessed 14 Nov 2018.

Valentin M. A., Ma S. L., Zhao A., Legay F. and Avrameas A. (2011) Validation of immunoassay for protein biomarkers: Bioanalytical study plan implementation to support pre-clinical and clinical studies. J Pharm Biomed Anal, 5, 869–877

Van Der Gugten J. G., Wong S. and Holmes D. T. (2016) Quantitation of Insulin Analogues in Serum Using Immunoaffinity Extraction, Liquid Chromatography, and Tandem Mass Spectrometry. Methods Mol Biol, 1378, 119–130

Van Eps A. W. and Pollitt C. C. (2006) Equine laminitis induced with oligofructose. Equine Vet J, 3, 203–208

Vick M. M., Adams A. A., Murphy B. A., Sessions D. R., Horohov D. W., Cook R. F., Shelton B. J. and Fitzgerald B. P. (2007) Relationships among inflammatory cytokines, obesity, and insulin sensitivity in the horse. J Anim Sci, 5, 1144–1155

Vick M. M., Sessions D. R., Murphy B. A., Kennedy E. L., Reedy S. E. and Fitzgerald B. P. (2006) Obesity is associated with altered metabolic and reproductive activity in the mare: effects of metformin on insulin sensitivity and reproductive cyclicity. Reprod Fertil Dev, 6, 609–617

Warnken T., Brehm R., Feige K. and Huber K. (2017) Insulin signaling in various equine tissues under basal conditions and acute stimulation by intravenously injected insulin. Domest Anim Endocrinol, 61,17–26

Warnken T., Reiche D., Huber K., Feige, K (2018) Comparison of endocrine and metabolic responses to oral glucose test and combined glucose-insulin tests in horses. Pferdeheilkunde, 34, 316–326

Warnken T., Schumacher S., Frers F., Delarocque J., Huber K., Feige K. (2018) Does naso-gastric tubing influence clinical relevant oral glucose test results?. 10th European College of Equine Internal Medicine Congress: 2–4 November, 2017. J Vet Int Med, 2, 878

Weeks I., Kricka L.J., Wild D. (2013) Signal generation and detection systems. In Wild D. (Ed): The Immunoassay Handbook: Theory and Applications of Ligand Binding, ELISA and Related Techniques. 4th Edition, Elsevier Science, Newnes, 267–285

Wilcox G. (2005) Insulin and insulin resistance. Clin Biochem Rev, 2, 19–39

Wild D. (2013) Immunoassay for Beginners. In Wild D. (Ed): The Immunoassay Handbook: Theory and Applications of Ligand Binding, ELISA and Related Techniques. 4th Edition, Elsevier Science, Newnes, 7–10

Wyse C. A., Mcnie K. A., Tannahill V. J., Murray J. K. and Love S. (2008) Prevalence of obesity in riding horses in Scotland. Vet Rec, 18, 590–591

Yakar S., Liu J. L. and Le Roith D. (2000) The growth hormone/insulin-like growth factor-I system: implications for organ growth and development. Pediatr Nephrol, 7, 544–549

Yalow R. S. and Berson S. A. (1959) Assay of plasma insulin in human subjects by immunological methods. Nature, 1648–16

14 ACKNOWLEDGEMENTS

I would particularly like to thank...

... **Prof. Dr. Karsten Feige** for excellent and continuous support through the last years. I am grateful for the opportunity to continue with my research on equine endocrinology. The opportunity to make up own ideas, realize projects and finalize studies to support the ongoing research in the rapidly growing field of research on equine insulin dysregulation.

... **Prof. Dr. Korinna Huber** for excellent education in scientific research, for infinite support on professional and especially metal level, taking time for inspiring discussions and motivation to carry on with equine endocrine related research always focusing on a strong combination of basic research and clinical relevant application.

Furthermore, I wish to thank...

... **Kathrin Hansen** for her help to "rescue all the fat ponies" and personal support in laboratory work at the Department of Physiology.

... **Svenja Schenzel, Claudia Schaub, Julien Delarocque, Florian Frers and Anne Grob** for the nice and constructive collaboration in our research group.

... my **colleagues at the Clinic for Horses**, who gave me the opportunity to finish the thesis despite a heavy workload.

... **Dr. Dania Reiche** and **Dr. Johanna Sonntag** for continues inspiring discussions, excellent support and constructive criticism.

Special thanks are directed to...

... my grandpa **Heinz Fliege** for continuous motivation to complete a doctorate, because a "PhD" is not a "Dr." – this is for you!

... **Kathrin**, my **family** and my **friends** for metal support and belief in me at any time.